Pedal, Stretch, Breathe

The Yoga of Bicycling

Kelli Refer

Pedal, Stretch, Breathe: The Yoga of Bicycling

Text and illustrations copyright 2013 Kelli Refer
Cover design by Joe Biel

Taking the Lane / Elly Blue Publishing—Portland, Oregon
www.takingthelane.com

A part of the contents of this book was originally published in 2012 as a zine with the same title.

First printing

Table of Contents

Welcome

Thank you so much for picking up a copy of *Pedal, Stretch, Breathe: The Yoga of Bicycling*. You don't have to define yourself as cyclist to ride a bike or think of yourself as a yogi to stretch and breathe. No carbon fiber bikes or pricey yoga pants are required here. In the ever growing industries of yoga and bicycles, it is my intention to bring you something that stems from my personal experiences of riding my bicycle and teaching yoga.

This book highlights key yoga poses that work with the needs of an everyday bike rider. While some people may have enough time to roll out their yoga mat and do a 15 minute yoga practice before heading to a meeting, I know many of you are too busy for that. That is ok. I am a big advocate of sneaking in a little bit of yoga in your day.

The Yoga of Bicycling isn't only physical, but also offers mental shifts, too. Bicycling has the capacity to shift the paradigm of the way you see and interact with where you live. Distance is transformed, community is redefined. Try to integrate the same mindfulness of a yoga practice into the act of riding a bike. See what happens. When you integrate a yoga perspective into your riding it amplifies the importance of the present moment and helps you listen to your body.

This book is structured like a yoga class. We introduce the basics at the beginning—finding your pedals, we call it here. Then we start to get moving, stretching it all out. It is in this section of the book that you will find yoga poses to practice before, during or after rides. The final section of the book is where we explore the cycles of breath, the seasons, and the chakras. This section closes with meditation. And naturally, we close the book with Savasana, or as other authors might call it, a conclusion.

Enjoy exploring your body, your breath and your bicycle!

Part 1

Foundations: Find your pedals

The importance of staying present

Riding a bicycle and doing yoga are both great ways to practice being present. Staying in tune with your body, mind, and breath just feels good, whatever you are doing, but especially with activities like these.

It takes practice to cultivate presence of mind. Our minds tend to fixate on the past, like when that jerk honked at you. Or we ponder the future, like wondering what is over the next hill. Yoga asks practitioners to, instead, stay in the body and watch the breath. On a bicycle, when we are aware of our body, our breath, and our surroundings we enhance our ability to adapt to the changing circumstances of the road. When we are aware and alert we are safer—both on our bikes and on our yoga mats.

In either activity, if you notice your mind starting to wander, it helps to bring your focus to your breath. Your breath is always present.

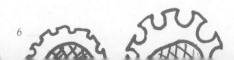

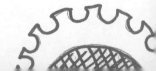

Yamas & Niyamas: The guiding principles of yoga and how they relate to bikes

Yoga mostly conjures images of people practicing Asana, the poses, and maybe the breathing and meditating, too. Beyond those things, there is a whole philosophical dimension of yoga that is less well known. One of the major historical texts of yoga is *The Yoga Sutras* by Patanjali, who is considered one of the major founders of yoga. He outlines an eight limbed path of yoga, offering guidelines for a meaningful life. The yamas and niyamas are the first two limbs of this path. The yamas offer sage advice on how to treat other people. The niyamas are more personal or spiritual practices to help you evolve. You might find that some of these principles speak more to you than others, which is just fine.

One way to work with yamas and niyamas is to pick one particular principle that inspires you or that you would like to invite into your life. Write the word on paper and stick it up somewhere prominent in your home. The visual reminder helps you stay connected with that idea. For instance, before I was going to move to Seattle I wrote down the word "aparigraha," which means non-hoarding, and posted it on the fridge. As I was packing it helped me remember to let go of the material things I didn't need for the next journey of my life.

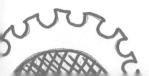
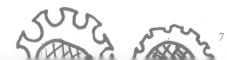

Yamas

Ahimsa ~ Non-Violence

The very first yama, or guiding principle for a yoga practice, is ahimsa, which translates to non-violence.

We often hear about or see violent interactions, and we know what they look like. Non-violence, though—what does that look like? At first we think of peaceful protestors, like Gandhi. But surely we see non-violence more often than that.

I have been keeping my eyes open for peaceful interactions. I've noticed that non-violent action is hidden in small acts of kindness like a simple smile or genuine hug, a moment of consideration for someone else, or a self-loving thought and kind words.

Some of the most violent encounters I have ever experienced have been on the road. Once I was turning left onto my street and a person in the car honked at me. So I flipped the person off (not the best move). This infuriated the driver, who decided to turn left and follow me and then cut me off by turning into a driveway to yell at me. A lot of very, very angry words were shared. I eventually just walked away. I was totally shaken up. My neighbors and friends nearby helped calm me down. It could have gone worse. Thankfully it didn't.

The really weird thing about biking is you never know what you are going to get. You may be riding down the street and get a friendly honk from a friend in a car or see another bike riding buddy and stop and chat. Or you might all of a sudden be dealing with some serious road rage.

We traverse these emotional encounters like we traverse the hills. It is part of the journey. If yoga has really taught me one thing, it is that to deal best with a situation you must be present, not reliving the past or planning the future. And if you want to access the present you need to focus on your breath.

One of things I am working on the road is de-escalating situations, taking it down a notch. Yelling back, which is often my gut reaction, does not always serve the situation best. Perhaps there is an element of forgiveness we all need to work on. We are human and we make mistakes on the road. I believe we will make fewer mistakes if we are present. We might even make more connections if we smile.

Satya ~ Truthfulness

We lie to ourselves all of the time, telling ourselves half truths and false stories. We insist that we are not strong enough to ride all the way to work or that we will never be able to touch our toes. But our personal truth changes and evolves, just like our bodies do. Lo and behold a few days, weeks, months, or years later we realize: Hey, I can do that. What I thought was true, that story I told myself for years, that was a lie.

One particular belief I held was that biking in the suburbs was really hard and dangerous. I spent my teenage years in Littleton, Colorado, where the car is king. While I biked on some trails in town, they didn't go directly to useful places, and I never took my bike out of our housing development. Even when I started biking while living in nearby Denver, when I went to see my parents a car was always involved. In my most recent visit, however, I ventured out into the streets and sidewalks to rediscover my hometown via bike. This was an incredibly liberating experience.

As a teenager, it never occurred to me that I could go places by bike. These recent outings were so enlightening because I realized the story I had told myself about biking in the suburbs was not true. Drivers passed us respectfully on the street, and I noticed more bike racks and other riders than I had in the past. While there are improvements that need to be made along major roads that would go along way to making cycling more accessible, for the first time it seemed possible to ride a bike for transportation in Littleton.

We live in a car culture. That is a current truth. But we can look at history to remind ourselves that the world once ran without cars. I'd like to think we can shift away from being so car oriented. I have come to realize that cars are not going to disappear completely. But as I bike on the road and create space for more folks to hop on their bikes and join me, we will transform our cities and towns. We are creating a bike movement that shifts us in a more sustainable direction. That is my truth.

Asteya ~ Non-Stealing

Don't steal other people's stuff and especially don't steal someone's bike—pretty straightforward, right? But our study of this precept can go beyond stealing in the material sense.

How important is your time? So often we are searching for more hours in the day. While bikes may not be able to travel at the same high speeds as cars on a highway, bikes can actually save us a lot of time. In many cases riding your bike is actually faster than taking the bus, and in rush hour traffic bikes often pass cars. Bikes navigate space in a more fluid way, by allowing you to take a shortcut through the park, for instance. Since bikes cost less than cars and have fewer costs like gas and insurance, you work fewer hours to pay for a bike. So go for a bike ride, and don't steal anymore precious time from yourself!

Let's look out from an even wider angle. When you choose to drive a car there are many hidden costs that are not accounted for in your checkbook. When you drive you are using resources like fuel, the materials needed to make and (one day destroy) cars, and all the resources used to make highways. When you drive, you contribute to pollution of the air and damage to roads and infrastructure. Space in the city is finite and cars take up a lot of that precious space. In the space of one car parking spot you can easily fit

16 bikes. The harsh costs of driving don't only take a toll on your wallet; all of society has to pay for them, and often it's the people who can't afford to drive that suffer the most.

Brahmacharya ~ Moderation

At times I can get a little yoga-ed out. I love practicing and teaching yoga. But I am not so much in love with a lot of the images that surround yoga culture of super flexible, skinny ladies advertising super expensive yoga clothing. Sometimes I need to take a break.[1]

But then I always remember—that isn't what yoga is about. Yoga is when we are real with ourselves and accept our body exactly as it is today. Yoga is a practice, and if we come back to it, there will continually be ups and downs, just like the terrain we ride our bikes over.

How can you tell if you have gone into the realm of excess with bicycling? Well, have you ever lectured someone at a party about the virtues of bicycling or do you give out unsolicited advice about new bike components? Or perhaps the once lively group conversation has shifted towards two gearheads comparing the latest cranksets, while everyone else stares at the wall. These are signs you may have fallen into the realm of excess or obsession. Bicycling is something to be passionate about, but try to leave the lectures and nitty-gritty chat alone. There is more to life than your daily yoga practice or finding the perfect bike part.

Brahmacharya is all about stepping back and looking at the bigger picture. We are lucky to have a great diversity of people on

1 One thing that helped me out of a yoga funk* was the book *21st Century Yoga: Culture, Politics, and Practice*. Suddenly I was reading about people who were expressing and writing critiques of yoga, while still being avid practitioners.

*That particular funk was caused almost exclusively by hearing about a line of designer meditation pants that cost $999.

this earth with a plethora of interests and passions. It is important to engage in your interests without totally letting them dominate your life.

Aparigraha ~ Non-Possessiveness

Take a breath in and then take a big exhale. Make whatever sound you need to get out of your system.

You just gotta let it go sometimes. Our breath is a great tool to help us access aparigraha. We need oxygen, so we inhale. Then we use what we need and exhale the rest to make room in our lungs for fresh air. This is the cycle of breath. If we don't ever let go of what we have we will never make room for anything new.

Aparigraha is a great yama to invoke when packing for a bike tour, when moving to a new place or trying to simplify your space to make room for your yoga mat. I must have talked a lot about aparigraha when my partner and I moved across the country because it is the one yama he knows about. After volunteering at the Bike Works, a non-profit in Seattle, he shared this story with me. He was working the Kids Bike Swap, an event that helps kids trade in their outgrown bikes for ones that fit them better. He was supervising kids in the test ride area. He observed that children had one of two reactions: Kids were either super excited to get a new bike or they were terribly sad to give away their old bike.

Tom was assisting one kid who was having a particularly hard time letting go of his bike. In trying to explain to the kid that only way to get a new bike that would be even better is to let go of the old one this line slipped out: "Aparigraha, dude."

There are a lot of things that we need to let go of. Sometimes it is actual, physical stuff, but even more often we need to let go of grudges, bad habits, and expectations. Remember to exhale, and the grip of whatever you are holding onto will surely loosen.

Niyamas

Saucha ~ Cleanliness

Bikes aren't too clean. My bike is almost always dirty. My fenders are coated in mud and most of my clothes have bike grease somewhere on them. There is something to be said about giving your bike a bath, at least once before winter and once in spring. Wiping away road grime will make your bike feel lighter, faster and little bit happier. There is this theory that if you keep your bike clean all of your components will be at optimal performance. If you clean your bike regularly, you can let me know if this theory pans out. In the meantime I will be riding through muddy puddles and getting bike grease on my new skirt.

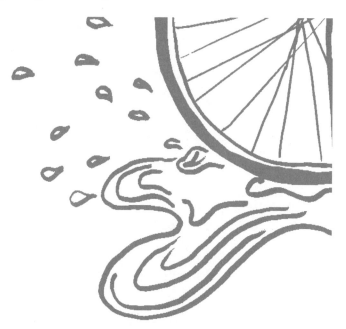

Santosha ~ Contentment

I love to say this word, santosha. It just rolls of the tongue so easily. Contentment is easily found on bike rides. There is so much bliss during an early morning commute, so early the stars are still out and the streets are calm and peaceful. Santosha is the contentment of becoming one with rain, the sounds on the pavement and the drops rolling down your cheeks. No matter the weather, enjoy the sensations of just biking, breathing and being.

The magical thing about contentment is that it can be summoned in almost any situation. Santosha is a practice, one that we are not always good at as a society that constantly tries to do more. It isn't that trying to achieve more is inherently bad—it often helps unveil our deepest potential. But practice being happy with where you are at. There is nothing wrong with you, nothing that needs fixing. You are a person, whole and complete with a wonderful spectrum of feelings and emotions.

Sometimes you will get a flat tire on the side of the road, sometimes you will fall out of your balance pose. You can still be content exactly where you are in your body and with your bike.

Tapas ~ Heat, Fire and Dedication

"It's about 1% physical and 99% spiritual" ~Rider on the Fargo Street Hill Climb in LA

Hills. They bring out a cyclist's tapas, or inner fire. I certainly know that the best way to warm up in winter is find the hilliest route to work and charge up that hill until the warmth spreads to fingers and toes.

We have all faced that one really big hill. The one that scared us. It looked too steep to even exist, let alone ride a bike up it. I faced one of those hills right after getting a cast removed from my right hand. It was a lovely Summer's day and a group of friends wanted to bike to Discovery Park, a forested park that has lovely beach by the Puget Sound. I was ready to get back into my regular riding routine and let go of my fear of falling. When we arrived at the park were at the top of a giant hill and wanted to get down by the water. I felt weak and out of shape, nervous to ride down such a large hill knowing that eventually I would have to bike back up it. But I longed to put my feet in the cold salt water, so I rode down anyway.

The tide was low, revealing a variety of hidden treasures and unique little creatures that live in the shallow tide pools. The sun was shining and I drank in all of the beauty of this wonderful place. After a while it was time to leave the sand and make our way home.

The hill was relentless. My heart pounded, my legs burned and I wanted to stop. But I kept breathing and pedaling, breathing and pedaling. I felt the heat in my body, the sweat dripping down my brow. I was going to make it. I had to keep going, keep pedaling and breathing. I was determined to do it...to make it up to the top and ride all the way home. I knew I could make it all the way up if could just keep riding. And I did. Climbing back up this hill was the process of reclaiming my power and letting go of my fear.

Svadhyaya ~ Self-study

Yoga is a potent practice for self-study. Take time to notice without judgement what you feel in your body. In the mornings your body may feel stiff. Take a moment to notice this, and then find a simple stretch or mat-free sun salutation so you can feel a little looser as you commute to work.

Get curious about yourself. What do you notice that you've never noticed before? Maybe your toes, where are they pointed? How about your forearms or the side of your body? When you practice a hip opener, is one side tighter than the other?

I have found that by importing the awareness I have on my mat, I pay more attention to my habits as I ride.

Not just physical habits, but my habitual thought patterns. I try to notice the alignment of my knees over the pedal and how I hold the handlebars.

Notice your thoughts, do you judge yourself harshly or get distracted easily? Try to watch the thoughts that drift in and out of your mind.

Noticing your habits is the way to get to know a part of yourself better. Try your best not to judge your habits as good or bad. Just notice them. Observe what you usually do and see if it serves you well. Some habits are helpful, like being extra mindful when you are making a left hand turn. Others may not be as helpful. When you bring awareness to your habits you are in a better position to change them if they do need changing. Finally, remember that you are more than your body, your habits and your mode of transit. Know you are far more than the sum of your parts.

Ishvara Pranidhana ~ Surrender

At the end of yoga class we practice savasana, or corpse pose, where you lay on the ground, still and silent. All of the effort of flowing from pose to pose is done. Effort makes way for ease.

All of your control and discipline have helped you access your power and inner strength, but at the end of the day it is time to give that up and practice surrender.

We've been trained to think surrender is for losers, that we should never give up, always keep fighting. But that isn't very sustainable. We don't need to bike up never ending hills.

The effort of the hill climb gives way to the ease to coasting downhill. Gravity pulls you closer to your destination. Speed increases and you feel air blow on your cheeks. There is little or no effort and almost the sensation of weightlessness. At times, surrender can be scary and you find yourself gripping the brakes to slow down and feel in control.

But what happens when you let go? Let go of the brakes, let go of the handle bars and soar down the hill. Let gravity do the work. Surrender happens when we abdicate total control and let the mysterious universe have her way with us.

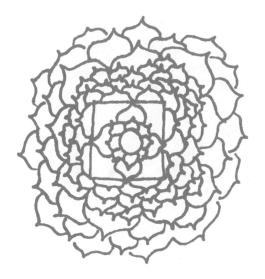

Taking a comfortable seat

Asana, the physical practice of yoga, is the third limb of yoga. It used to refer to all of the yoga postures, but the word asana itself translates to "a comfortable seat." Many of the yoga postures are challenging but we practice finding ease and contentment amidst the effort. In this section I offer tips to find your comfortable seat on your mat and on your bike. So go on, hop in saddle and ride with ease, no matter what the hill ahead looks like.

Here are some pointers to finding your comfortable seat. The lotus indicates a yoga exercise and the wrench a bike-based action.

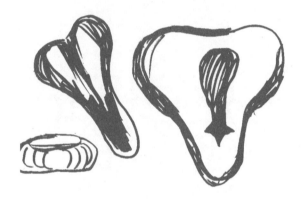

Start from the ground up. Notice your feet all the way to your head

 Which direction are your toes pointing? How about you knees and then hips, shoulders and head? When setting up a yoga pose do a scan from your feet to your head. See how your body feels. You will notice if you move your foot that starts to impact where knees and hips go.

Begin to notice what is happening from pedal to helmet. Notice the balls of the feet push into the pedal. If you have toe clips, feel the pull and push dynamic.

Notice the alignment of your bones and major joints—your knees, hips shoulders and wrists

 Move slowly so you have time to pay attention to your alignment. One of the things I see most in yoga class is a misguided knee in lunges. When you are in a lunge if your knee bends beyond your ankle, your feet need to be farther apart, so the knee stacks directly over the ankle. Knees also tend to lean in towards the big toe side of your foot. Again, bring your knee back over your ankle.

 Are your knees over your ankles? At times this may require making minor changes to your saddle position and handle bars. Frame geometry varies a lot from one bicycle to another. It is important that you find a frame that fits your body. You should be able to stand over the the top tube with your feet comfortably grounded.

Let your shoulders relax.

 Shoulders seem to involuntarily creep up towards the ears, contracting the muscles in the upper back and neck. Most of the time we don't actually need to engage these muscles, so remember to slide your shoulders down your back. This especially important to remember in Chair Pose.

 Next time you are riding, check in with your shoulders. Are they reaching up by your ears? Are you hunched over or more upright? Slide your shoulders down your back, this will give you a more assertive posture and facilitates deep breathing.

Pay attention to your hands. There are 26 bones in each hand (more or less...we are all a little different), including seven in your wrist, which gives humans great dexterity.

Notice the natural curl of your fingers when you hands are relaxed by your side. Experiment with different hand gestures or mudras, to see how that changes your pose. One of my favorite mudras is Anjali Mudra, where both hands are in prayer position with thumbs touching your sternum at heart center. This is a great place to check in with your heartbeat and breathing. It can also be a great way to end a yoga practice.

Keep as much weight out of your hands as possible when you bike. Circle wrists every so often. Wave to other people and use your hands to help communicate where you are riding to other road users. Sometimes I find it helpful to point to people exactly where I am going. When people are very rude it can be really tempting to make other not so friendly gestures...but that seldom improves the road rage situation. Folks tend to grip the handlebars hard when they are nervous about traffic or road conditions. So just be aware if you are feeling stressed. Try to breathe and relax and then ease up on your grip.

Use your vision!

You can use your eyes to check alignment in yoga class. When doing yoga outside remember to take in the sights. Notice the sky, the horizon and the small things under your feet. Sometimes closing your eyes enables you to tap into the feeling of your body or pay more attention to your other senses.

Peripheral vision is important for scoping out traffic and noticing cool street graffiti. To increase your field of vision try this exercise: Gently turn your head to the left and right noticing how far you can see. Then turn your head to the left but look right and then switch. Repeat slowly twice more on each side. Then look to the left, look to the right and see if your vision has expanded! Reminder, do this when you are not riding your bike.

Everything changes

The pose that was easy three months ago may have become the hardest thing to do in the world today. That is ok.

Notice how changes in traffic and landscape affect how you feel. Our comfort level changes depending on where we are on our streets and in our bodies and minds.

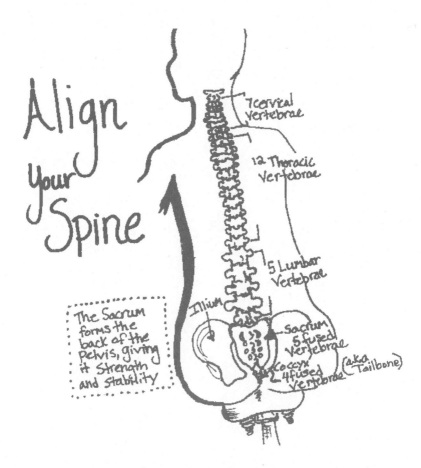

Align Your Spine

7 cervical Vertebrae

12 Thoracic Vertebrae

5 Lumbar Vertebrae

Ilium

Sacrum 5 fused Vertebrae

Coccyx 4 fused Vertebrae (aka Tailbone)

The Sacrum forms the back of the Pelvis, giving it Strength and Stability

Letting Go of the Mat

About six years ago, when I lived in Colorado, I bought a really lovely biodegradable yoga mat. I was so excited to upgrade to a less toxic mat. But after less than two years of consistent use, both indoors and out, my biodegradable mat started to biodegrade.

First it was just a little stretch here, or a little chunk missing over there. Then one day, I was doing yoga in the desert and my little mat bit the dust. I guess I should have seen that coming.

Ever since then I have been mat free.

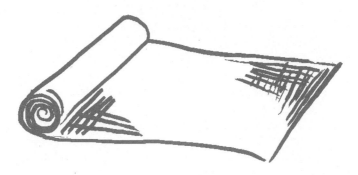

Just kidding.

I actually do still use a mat at studios. But I am not really attached to "my yoga mat." Indoors the yoga mat provides a safe space to explore and its grip helps me stay put in standing poses. Outdoors, though, I love the feeling grass below my feet and hands, even if it makes me sneeze! I also love practicing in peculiar spots, like on my bicycle.

Getting off the mat fosters presence and awareness. You notice the subtle shifts in the ground below. You shut your eyes and hear what is happening in the world around you. Balancing is especially elusive when you are outside with the wind moving things around and an uneven ground below your feet.

You do not need fancy or special equipment to practice yoga or ride a bicycle. In fact, when we step outside of the comfort zone those products provide, our awareness and presence increases.

Slowing Down

It's okay to slow down.

We live in a culture saturated with big egos where we are encouraged to go faster and push harder all the time. This kind of constant struggle to become better, faster, slimmer, etc., can really drive our bodies and spirits into the ground. In most cases I find yoga and cycling to be incredibly nourishing and healing activities. But when ego steps in and drives us to beyond our limit it can result in injury.

We all have an edge, where you can bike just a little faster or go a little deeper into your lunge. The edge is a great place to be. Just like the tide, your edge ebbs and flows with your energy. I like to emphasize that that rest is good for you. Even riding a bike slowly you will make it to where you need to go. It is okay to give yourself permission to do what is best for your body every single day.

Some days we need a restorative twist. Other days we need sprints up the hill. Give yourself permission to do what honors your body best.

Part 2

Stretch It Out:
Before and After
Your Ride

Static vs. Dynamic Stretching

Static stretching is where you take a pose and hold it. This stretch can be active, like when you contract one group of muscles to stretch the opposite group of muscles. For example, you engage the quads in your down dog pose so that you can stretch the Hamstrings. You can also have passive stretching, where you put in minimal effort and simply let gravity do the work. Check out the restorative section of poses that use props to support you in passive stretching.

Dynamic stretching is where you move through several poses sequentially. This is a great way to warm up your body. Move with your breath between the poses in this section and make your own sequences.

Find Your Flow: Creating a Warm-Up Ritual

I have found that if, before you set out on your bike, you take just one whole minute to gather your things and your thoughts and check in with your breath, you will carry with you a sense of ease and awareness on your commute.

If you have a few extra minutes in your day, a small warm up routine before you ride will help you stay even more present. Even two or three minutes of stretching makes all the difference to your muscles. Not only will your body feel a little better, but your mind will be prepared for the road ahead.

There is a lot of evidence to support this idea. Social psychologist Amy Cuddy gives a wonderful TED Talk on what she calls "Power Poses," postures that make you feel expansive and take up space. Research shows that just two minutes of practicing power poses increases a measurable hormonal change, boosting testosterone and lowering the stress hormone cortisol, and that this results in increased confidence.

Cuddy's studies were related to job interviews, but the same principle applies for riding your bike. The road is a shared social space. When you ride there, confidence helps you be more safe and comfortable there, especially when you need to take the lane.

The following yoga poses are power poses that should serve the same purpose. This handy dandy flow chart will help you develop a routine that works for you. Just like those quizzes in teen magazines that help you figure out your style, the chart helps you find your flow.

Start simple with a pose or two. Our bodies' needs evolve day by day, so see what feels good and experiment. Modifications you might like to try are in parentheses.

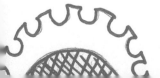
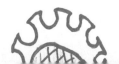

Pre-Ride Flow Chart

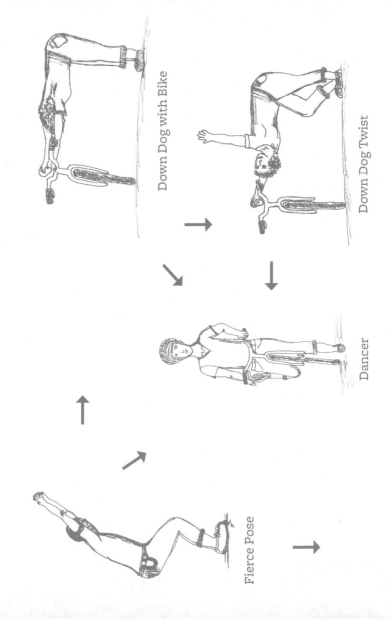

Down Dog with Bike

Down Dog Twist

Dancer

Fierce Pose

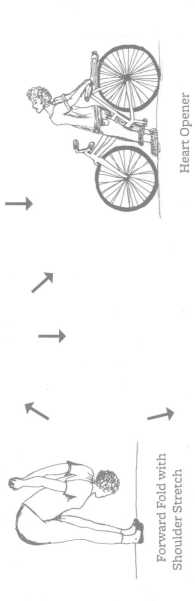

Heart Opener

Forward Fold with
Shoulder Stretch

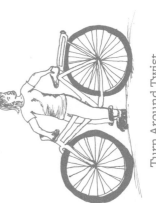

Turn Around Twist

Sample flows

- Fierce pose → Dancer →
  Standing Bike Twist

- Down-Dog w/ Bike → Down Dog Twist →
  Heart Opener

Fierce Pose a.k.a. Chair Pose: Utkatasana

Strengthens core and quads and builds heat in your body. If your knees hurt after you ride, using this pose to strengthen your quads will help take stress off your joints.

- Feet are hip distance apart and parallel facing forward
- Bend your knees and sit hips back as if sitting in a chair
- Check the alignment of your knees: make sure they are right your toes rather than collapsing towards each other
- Engage your core. Your low belly hugs up and in towards your spine
- Raise your arms above your head, with pinkies facing forward
- Slide your shoulders down your back, away from your ears

(Variation: Try this pose with arms parallel to the ground, palms facing down and to build ankle strength, try it on your tip toes)

Down Dog with Your Bike: Adho Mukha Svanasana

A wonderful pose to stretch out the backs of the legs and open the shoulders

- Stand facing the side of your bike holding on to the saddle and handlebars (Variation: place your hands on the top tube shoulder distance apart)
- Step back until your torso is parallel to the ground
- Your ears should be framed by your biceps. This keeps your neck in line with the rest of your spine
- Feet are hip distance apart, with toes facing your bike
- Knees are bent just a little. You can also bend one knee and stretch the other calf

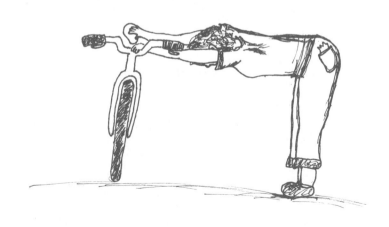

Down Dog Twist: Parivrtta Adho Mukha Svanasana

Opens tight hips and shoulders plus a detoxifying spinal twist

- Start at your bike in Down Dog
- Bend right knee, keep left leg straight
- Inhale, Extend your left arm up to the sky
- Exhale twist from the center of your ribs
- Gaze towards the clouds if that feels ok in your neck
- Release and switch sides.

Continue side to side if you like, inhaling to lift one arm up, exhale releasing, inhale switching sides to flow with your breath. This stretches your IT band and outer hips

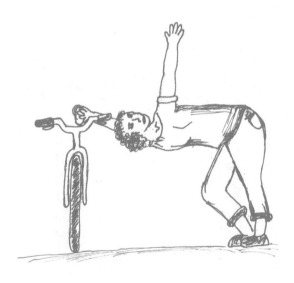

Dancer's Pose: Natarajasana

This elegant pose opens the front of your body and develops balance with your bike plus gives a stretch your quadriceps

- Straddle your bike, shifting weight to right side and root down
- Hold your brake with your right hand, Engage your core for stability
- Bend your left knee and grab your foot
- Pull your foot into your butt to open tight hip flexors and quads, breathe
- Kick your foot into your hand to open your shoulder
- Remember to switch sides

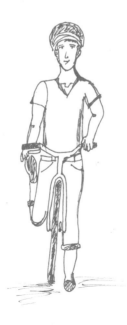

Forward Fold with Shoulder Stretch: Uttanasana

Gently open your hamstrings, low back and heart.

- Stand with feet parallel and hip distance
- Interlace fingers behind your back, pull arms behind you
- Squeeze your shoulders together
- Hinge at your hips to fold forward, keep a micro-bend in your knees
- Slide shoulders up the line of the back
- Release arms from behind your back and let them hang loosely (Or interlace your fingers behind your neck, allow your elbows to hang heavily by your ears. This is a great release for a stiff neck)
- Shift the weight into the front of your feet, wiggle your toes
- Relax your head, shake it "no" and nod your head "yes"
- Let go of any tension in your neck & face
- Slowly roll up vertebrae by vertebrae and let your head come up last

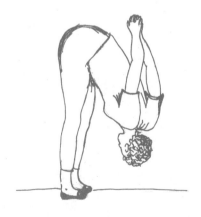

Heart Opener

Your bike makes excellent support for this lovely chest opener. Also a great pose to do at rest stops on long rides.

- Standing over your bike, grab the saddle behind you
- Keep your low belly engaged, transverse abdominal
- Lift your sternum to the sky
- Slide your shoulders down your back to support your heart
- Breathe into the front of your body and into your arms
- Gaze up to the sky and assess the accuracy of the weather forecast

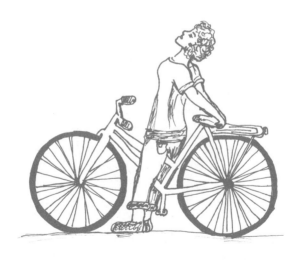

Turn Around Twist

Long stoplight? No problem. Add lift to your twist to check out what is going on behind you.

- Stand over your bike, feet forward
- Inhale, reach the crown of your head up to the sky
- Exhale, twist from the center of your ribs
- Use your saddle and handlebars for leverage in your twist
- Twist to the other side for balance
- Smile at everyone sharing the road with you!

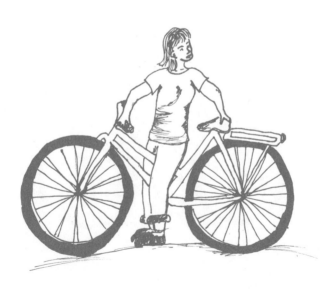

When You Arrive

Take a moment to appreciate where you have ridden. Enjoy putting your feet on the ground and take a simple standing pose or two.

Wide Legged Forward Fold: Prasarita Padottanasana

This is a great pose for stretching out the legs. There is a lot of room to play with this pose finding different arm variations.

- Step your feet out wide with your toes pointing forward
- Hands can be at your hips or fingers interlaced behind your back
- Hinge at your hips finding a forward fold
- Keep a slight bend in your knees
- Allow your weight to shift to the big toe and pinky toe mounds at the front of your feet with wiggle room for toes

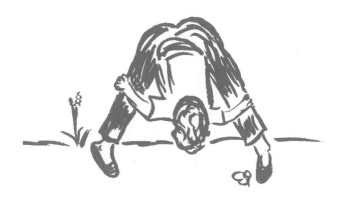

Figure Four: Eka Pada Utkatasana

- Start standing and shift your weight onto the left foot
- Slightly bend your knees
- Lift your right foot off the ground and rest the ankle just above your left knee
- Flex your right foot to protect your knee
- You may bring hands to heart center or hold onto your bike
- Hinge the hips and fold until you feel the stretch

This is a great rest stop stretch. You can even use your bike to aid your balance. This pose helps externally rotate the hip, helping you access the deep rotator muscles in your hip joint. More superficially, the pose opens up the glutes.

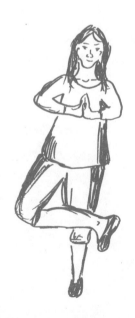

Part 3

Stretch It Out:
Build Your Wheel

Building Wheels in Bodies & Bicycles

I am enchanted by the beautiful mandala pattern of a bicycle's spokes. Mandala, a Sanskrit word, loosely translates to "circle." Mandala images are used in visual meditation. The bicycle wheel is a beautiful example of this form.

The first time I built a bicycle wheel it dawned on me that the process is similar to building the full wheel position on the mat. Urdhva Dhanurasana (Full Wheel) requires a delicate balance between effort and ease to find the perfect tension that holds your body in a strong, limber arch.

A yoga practice that emphasizes back bends can be especially useful for cyclists who ride with drop down handle bars or carry heavy backpacks. One of the key elements of the backbend is warming up—you must create space in the spine before lifting up into the full pose. Your backbend will not be helpful, and can cause injury, if you crunch your lumbar vertebrae together. When I am planning a yoga class that features wheel or bridge I warm up students by opening and strengthening shoulders, and lengthening the spine.

When truing wheels, at times it feels like you are not really making any changes. As I learned this art, I was constantly wondering if things were really improving. Similarly, the sphinx pose is a really easy back bend; when you do it, you are not sure if anything is happening. But yoga teaches us that subtle adjustments have a rippling effect that transforms whole postures. When preparing for full wheel, if you create that extra length in your spine, you find deeper backbends because there is more space between the vertebra. When truing wheels, a quarter turn in the wrong direction affirms that each little twist of nipple has its consequences.

Patience proved to be the biggest challenge for me in truing a wheel. Likewise, for many yoga practitioners patience is a challenge for moving into advanced postures.

Whenever I started to get really irritated or stuck while working on my wheel, I returned my focus to my breath. I advocate practicing ujjayi breath on and off the mat during challenging tasks. Ujjayi translates to "be victorious" or "to conquer." Breathe in and out of your nose, there is a gentle constriction in the back your throat and you hear a wave-like sound. This breath slows down and deepens breathing to increase oxygen intake and focus.

It took me awhile to really get a grasp on what I was doing with wheels, but once I gained a little bit of muscle memory and focus, I found my truing groove.

Remember to take your time and listen to your body about what feels good. Attending regular yoga classes supports the strength and flexibility of your spine. If this pose is very challenging, ask a teacher to help.

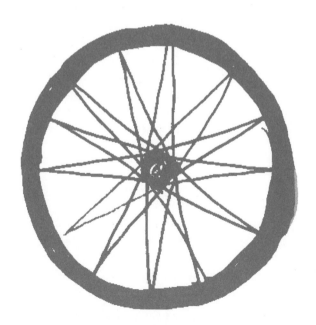

Building Your Wheel

Here are a series of postures that will help you work towards the goal of the Full Wheel. No need to hurry or rush things. It's possible to hurt your back by doing wheels too soon or too quickly, so take it nice and slow.

First, warm up! Grab your yoga mat or blanket (on a non-slip surface) and go into some Sun Salutations.

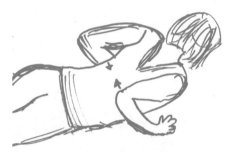

Low Cobra, part of the Sun Salutation.
(Squeeze elbows towards each other)

Sun Salutations

- Begin in Tadasana: Standing at the top of your mat toes facing forward
- Inhale reach arms up overhead, lifting up to create space in your spine
- Exhale take a forward fold, Uttanasana (tight hamstrings or sore low back? remember to bend your knees a little in your forward fold)
- Inhale to lift your torso half-way until you're parallel to the floor, looking at the ground with a flat back, Ardha Uttanasana

- Exhale fold into forward fold
- Plant both hands under the shoulders and step back to plank, or the top of a push up pose, *Dandasana*
- You may drop knees to the ground or not, but as you lower from your plank to your belly, keep your elbows hugging in by your sides
- Inhale peel your heart off the mat for Low Cobra, Bhujangasana
- Exhale curl your toes under and press back to Downward Facing Dog
- Take a big breath and repeat your Salutation 2 to 7 times
- Remember to move with your breath

Chair Pose, a.k.a. Fierce Pose: Utkatasana

- In Utkatasana take both hands to your knees with fingers facing each other and practice Cat/Cow and repeat for several rounds
- Then take a forward fold and step back to Down Dog, from there to High Plank, and finally back to lying on your belly.

Next is your Sphinx.

Sphinx: Salamba Bhujangasana

- The arms make a right angle, the elbows are bent right under the shoulder and the forearms are grounded; spread fingers wide
- Gently lift and lower lower your chin to relax your neck or cervical spine
- Notice where your back is bending in this pose- you are looking for the bend in the thoracic spine, or mid back. This is the least flexible part of the spine that we are trying to open in our

backbends

- Lower back to your belly and take a moment to rest. Breathe

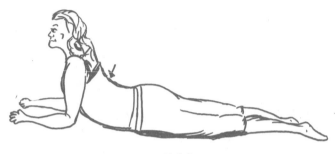

Sphinx
(Back bend originates from the mid-back)

Dancer: Natarajasana (on the floor)

- From your belly slide right arm out in front of your, reach out far to lengthen your spine and roll onto your right side
- Bend your left knee and capture your left foot with your left hand
- To get the great quad stretch here pull your heel into your butt
- To get the deeper backbend, start to kick your foot into your hand
- Try to relax your head on the bicep of your right arm
- Then practice on the other side one side might feel very different from the other

Bridge pose, Setu Bandha

Instructions for Bridge are on page 73. This is an essential step in building up to your Wheel. It can be done with or without a block.. Please feel free to work with bridge for as long as you'd like before even attempting wheel. Listen to your spine, not your ego, on how far to go.

Full Wheel Pose a.k.a. Upward Facing Bow: Urdhva Dhanurasana

- Begin on your back, as if doing Bridge
- Place your hands on the ground with fingers pointing towards your shoulders
- Begin to lift up into Bridge Pose
- Keep the elbows bent and squeezing towards each other- this stabilizes your shoulder girdle- Press your hands into the ground to start to lift hips up (Some people stop for a moment on their head before lifting all the way up, others do not)
- The trapezius will contract, helping lift your torso
- Keep your biceps squeezing in towards each other
- When in full wheel breathe and stay in the pose as long or a little as you'd like.
- Slowly lower down vertebrae by vertebrae

Attending a yoga class and letting the teacher know you would like to work on wheel is a great way to get added support and help into this advanced posture.

Cool Down Twist

Cool down with whatever twist pose you like best. Twists neutralize your spine after a large backbend, such as wheel

- Choose your favorite twist on your back, maybe both legs are bent and fall to one side while you gaze the opposite direction
- Breathe all the way down to your tailbone and up to the crown of your head
- Switch sides

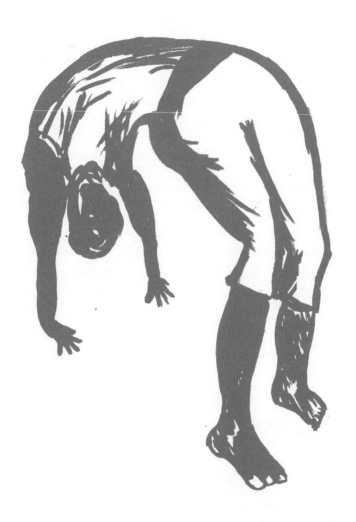

Part 4

Know Your Body:
Bicycling Muscle Groups and How to Stretch Them

Getting to Know Your Body Better

Any physical movement offers you wealth of information about your body. Yoga encourages you to acknowledge that information through svadhyaya, self-study. Anatomy is one way to deepen that self-study.

There are many fascinating intricacies of human anatomy, but for the sake of scope, I'll focus on major muscle groups that are particularly relevant for cyclists. It is also important to remember that your muscles do not act alone. We have tendons that help connect muscles to bone and ligaments that connect bone to bone. And of course that is just looking at the musculoskeletal system, let alone the nervous or endocrine or any other system of the body.

When we talk about anatomy, the "origin" of the muscle is where the muscle begins. The origin is closer to the trunk of the body, or proximal. Some muscles, like the biceps femoris of the hamstrings, have two origins. The "insertion" is where the muscle ends and is distal, closer to the hands and feet.

In every movement we take, the muscle that does most of the action is called the "agonist" or "prime mover." Muscles that play a supporting role are called "synergists." The muscle that counters the main action is called the "antagonist."

Think Newton, here. Every action must have an equal and opposite reaction:

"The antagonist produces the opposite action about a joint. For example, the quadriceps (at the front of the thigh) are the antagonists to the hamstrings when you flex your knee. When you extend your knee, the quadriceps are agonists and the hamstrings are the antagonists."

From *The Key Muscles of Yoga*, by Ray Long MD, a wonderfully illustrated technical guide to helping you learn the anatomy of many yoga poses.

Major Players in Pedal Power: Hamstrings and Quadriceps

The hamstrings and the quadriceps are in this constant dance as you pedal. On the top of the pedal, when the knee is bent the hamstrings are contracted and the quadriceps are lengthening. Then you push down, contracting the quads and lengthen the hamstrings. Then you engage the hamstrings to pull the pedal back to the top and the cycle continues.

In my own body, my hamstrings can feel so tight and limiting. I notice this especially as I take Downward Facing Dog with my bike or after a long day of running errands around town. It takes a long time to stretch out hamstrings and quads. You are trying to open an entire muscle group, and you don't want to just stretch the most superficial muscles. This is why your yoga teacher makes you stay in that pose about five more breaths than you would really like to.

Hamstrings

The hamstrings are the group of three major muscles that make up the majority of the back of the thigh: Biceps femoris, semitendinosus and semimembranosus. (Don't worry, there will not be a test on that.) They connect the sitting bones with the back of the knee, in a nice interwoven pattern.

Cycling strengthens the hamstrings, which is great, but to balance that strength you need to stretch to maintain flexibility. Tight hamstrings can cause low back pain and are more prone to injury. Stretching your hamstrings helps you find that balance of strength and flexibility.

Our hamstrings have a lot to teach us about patience. Move slowly and feel free to hold poses for a while, steadily breathing. Remember not to force hamstrings open, that could lead to injury. Be sweet to yourself, be sweet to your hamstrings.

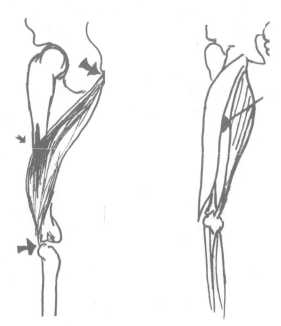

Hamstrings (view from back of body)
L: Biceps Femoris (top arrows show origins, at sitting bone and femur; bottom arrow shows insertion at tibia)
R: Semimembranosus (in between the other two hamstring muscles)

Some yoga poses that are especially good for stretching hamstrings: Downward Dog with Bike will especially open the Biceps Femoris. Reclining Big Toe Pose with a bungee will open the Semitendinosus and Semimembranosus. Restorative poses for the hamstrings include Legs up the Wall and Forward Fold with a block.

Remember to stay in the restorative postures for a little while, to slowly and gently stretch the back of your legs.

Quadriceps

The quadriceps are a group of four muscles that run along the front of the thigh. In cycling our quads are the main source of our pedal power. The quadriceps act by extending the leg from a bent knee to an extended leg. This is the primary action that propels us on pedals. Often cyclists have incredibly developed quads. It is important to give your quads a little bit of extra attention after a long haul, especially when you have been carrying heavy cargo or hitting the hills.

When you practice Fierce Pose, also known as Chair (page 30), you warm up your quadriceps while strengthening them. Strong quads also help keep your knees healthy. For a deep quad stretch check out the lovingly named Ninja Death Pose in English, or in sanskrit as *Eka Pada Rajakapotasana 2* on page 78.

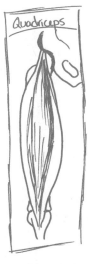

(*front view*)

The Tight Stuff: IT Band, Tensor Fascia Latae, Gluteus Maximus

Sometimes the everyday bike rider can't exactly pinpoint what it is that is all tight and sore and stuff, but it is generally around the hips. The repetitive motion of cycling can perpetuate tightness in the hips. The ball-in-socket hip joint was designed for strength and stability, which is great—until we lose flexibility.

The iliotibial band, more commonly called the IT band, is made of thick fibrous connective tissue (fascia) that runs on the outer edge of the leg.

The tensor fascia lata is a muscle that connects the iliac crest, the bony protrusions on the front of the pelvis to the IT band, helping lift the leg.

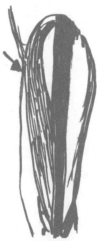

Side view of the hip and leg. The dark stripe is the IT band. The arrow points to the tensor fascia lata

The gluteus maximus is the most superficial of the butt muscles. It connects the back of the pelvis to the IT band, assisting with moving the knee.

Remember, it takes at least three minutes for fascia to stretch, so holding poses for longer periods of time will be more effective.

To lengthen the front of your body, try Dancer Pose, particularly the variation where you lay on your right side, resting your ear on your right arm. Then bend your left knee to catch your foot with your left hand. Breathe down the front of your body and remember to do the other side.

To get into the glutes try Reclined Pigeon on page 76. Or do the standing version called Figure Four on page 38, where you balance on one leg with a slight bend in the knee and rest the other ankle over the knee making the shape of a 4 with your legs.

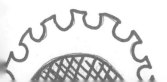
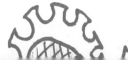

Adductor Magnus & Adductor Group

This group of muscles helps squeeze the thighs towards each other and is a synergist to the glutes. When we contract the Adductors we draw the energy of the legs towards each other and up towards the trunk, which can be particularly helpful when exploring wheel pose on page 54. To help open up the legs try a Wide Legged Forward Fold.

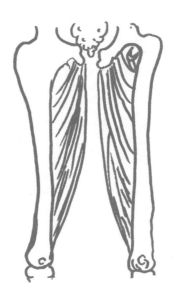

Adductor magnus (rear view), connects the sitting bones to the inside of the femur.

Psoas & Hip Flexors

The psoas (pronounced so-AHZ) is a wonderfully mysterious muscle that is nestled deep in your trunk. In fact, it is the deepest muscle in your body. In simple terms we rely on the psoas to keep us upright. This muscle is very intricately connected to our nervous system. It is responsible for our "gut feelings" and is connected to our survival instincts.

It is the only muscle that connects the spine to the legs. The psoas originates around where the thoracic spine meets the lumbar spine moving towards the pelvic basin. It inserts around the top of the femur. The iliacus is the muscle that fans out on the inside of the ilium (the pelvis). These two muscles are often grouped together and called the iliopsoas complex because they inform each other so much.

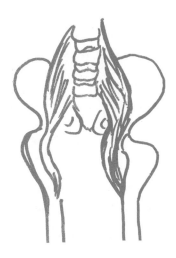

Front view of the psoas major and minor

The hip flexors as a group are the iliopsoas, the rectus femoris (of the quads), the sartorius (the longest muscle in the human body) and the tensor fascia latae and the adductor group (group that makes up the inner thigh). The hip flexors lift the leg for every rotation.

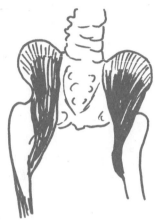

Front view of the illiacus

Restorative stretching alleviates tension around your pelvis. A tight psoas can be the source of pain, stifled breathing or poor digestion. When you relax your psoas and hip flexors you will feel revitalized and refreshed and able to better connect with your instincts.

I've included a lunge and twist to help you access your psoas and gently stretch your hip flexors. Fallen tree (next page) is great for relaxing the psoas. For a restorative pose that releases the hip flexors try Supported Bridge on page 73.

I found myself fascinated by the psoas and iliacus. If you want to learn more about this muscle, I highly recommend checking out *The Psoas Muscle* by Liz Koch.

Fallen Tree

This pose is best on a lazy morning, when you are feeling sleepy.

- Lay on your belly in bed or a sleeping bag
- Slide your left foot up your right leg for fallen tree pose
- Your left hip might lift up, that is a sign your psoas needs this pose
- Remember to switch sides

Low Lunge: Anjaneyasana

A basic pose to stretch your hips:

- Step the right foot to the front of your mat with the ankle aligning over the knee at a 90 degree angle, drop the left knee to the ground
- Press your heel into the mat and bring your hands to press on your thigh
- Shift your hips forward and lift chest up inviting length from tailbone up to the crown of your head
- Gently rock back and forth on the heel of the front foot to open up the front and and breathe into your hip flexors on the left side of your body
- Squeeze both legs energetically towards each other to increase stability
- Lift arms to the air
- Breathe down the left side of your body
- Repeat on the lunge on the second side

Mermaid Twist

This shape of this pose reminds me of a mermaid perching on a rock, gazing at the sea.

- Begin in a seated with your feet and sittings bones grounded
- Gently let your knees fall to the left, with the knees still bent place the left foot on the right thigh
- Most of your weight is on the left hip
- Press your fingertips into the ground to help lift up your torso up, creating more space between your vertebrae
- As you exhale deepen your twist
- Take your gaze behind you, peering over your shoulder, maybe you can see your other foot
- Remember to do the other side

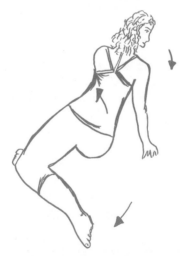

The mermaid twist originates from the mid-back. Gaze over your shoulder to look for your toes.

Trapezius: The Upper Back

Bike riders with drop down bars have most likely experienced some tension in the upper back and neck, this is due to tightness in the trapezius. The trapezius is a large trapezoidal shaped, superficial muscle on the back that connects the back of the skull and the shoulders and tapers down the back. It is the primary muscle involved in the "shrugging" of the shoulders. It is important to relax your shoulders, sliding the scapula (shoulder blade) down your back as you ride. I advise against carrying heavy backpacks or messenger bags. Grab a bike rack with a crate or a basket to help you carry things more comfortably and protect your upper back from chronic pain.

If upper back pain is a persistent problem as you ride, there is a chance that your bike is a little too long for you and you are constantly reaching too far forward, straining your neck and shoulders. Slide your seat forward or try different handlebars to see if those adjustments make your bike more comfortable for you.

To gently release some tension in the neck lean your ear over to your shoulder and gently nod your head, then slowly roll your chin to center and then over to the other side. Relax your jaw by separating your back teeth. Another great way to counteract the rounding of your upper back to spend some time in the Restorative Heart Opener on page 74.

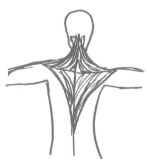

Cat/Cow in Chair

One of my favorite warm-ups when I only have one minute before I need to start pedaling if I want to make it to yoga class on time is Cat/Cow. This is also a great way to offer relief to your trapezius.

1. Bend your knees and sink your hips into an imaginary chair
2. Take you hands on your thighs and have your fingers facing each other
3. Inhale, send your heart forward and gaze up for Cow Pose
4. Exhale, round your back and look into your belly
5. Move back and forth between these poses with your breath

The same Cat/ Cow pose you can take in a chair is also accessible on your bicycle. This movement is especially nice in the middle of a long ride, and will provide a relief to your spine.

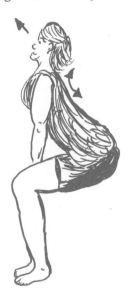 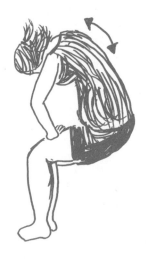

Calf Muscles

The calf muscle's main roles are to flex the foot and bend the knee. The origin of the gastrocnemius is through a tendon on the back of the femur and inserts halfway through the back of of the leg and meets up the with fibrous achilles tendon at the back of the heel. The soleus is a flat muscle that runs below the gastrocnemius. In our cycle of the pedal, the calf pull the heel up allowing you to bend the knee, then your quads kicks and you push forward.

A little stretch for the calf with your pedal

Many bike riders quickly learn this easy way to stretch tights calves on your bicycle. Stand up and let your heel dip below the pedal, lengthening the gastrocnemius and soleus muscles that make up the calf. This is a great tip for whenever you need a little change of pace or want to coast a bit and change your position.

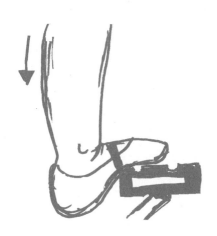

Core

People love it or hate core exercises, but no matter what we all have to use our core muscles.

In my teacher training program, there was a heavy emphasis on core strengthening. As someone who initially fell in love with yoga for its moments of stretched out bliss, core was never my favorite part. But six months later I was teaching my first regular class, twice weekly at a community center, and one of my regular students starts requesting core at the beginning of every class. This was a great way for me as a teacher to start integrating a variety of core strengthening into my yoga sequences that went beyond your typical sit-ups.

There is this notion that a lean "six-pack" of abs is the ideal of core strength, but that is really just the rectus abdominus showing off. Core strength is truly improved by focusing deeper, going into the center of your strength rather than the surface. The External Obliques move diagonally downward. The Internal Obliques move diagonally upward and aid in any twisting motions. The transverse abdominis is the deepest layer and runs laterally across the belly, like an internal belt that holds all your insides together. When you are using your deep core strength you will be able to maintain stamina to ride longer. Strengthening your core also supports your low back.

Notice if you wiggle from side to side as you ride. If you do, this is an indication you need to strengthen your transverse abdominis, the deepest of all abdominal muscles. (It might also be a sign that your seat is too high.) Hug your low belly up and in towards the spine—this stabilizes your torso and drops your focus into your lower body. Using your core as you ride supports your lower back and keeps hips healthy. It is also a way to access your inner power.

Uddiyana Bandha

Just about two fingers below your belly button, deep in your core, is the abdominal lock, or bandha. Engage the bandha by pulling your navel up towards the ribs and in towards the spine. When engaged during a yoga practice, the bandha creates a deeper sense of stability. Physiologically it is where many nerves branch out from the spinal cord going down to the legs and feet. This place is a source of our physical power.

When you need an extra boost because you are still a few miles away from where you are going, use your core. Know that there is a deep well of strength inside your core to draw on when you need it. And as always...remember to breathe.

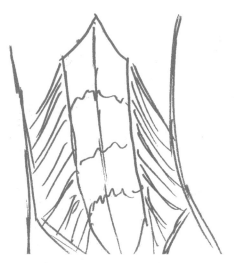

Obliques and rectus abdominus

Table Top

- Place hands under your wrists with fingers spread wide apart
- Knees are right under your hips
- Pull your lower belly (right below the belly button) up toward the ribs and towards the spine - this activates your core muscles and will help you be more stable
- Lift up one hand and reach it out in front of you for a hand-shake, pinky side of the hand towards the ground
- Extend the opposite leg back with the toes turned towards the grounds
- Imagine your foot is pressing on a wall, use the strength in your legs to reach way out through the fingers tips, you grow about an inch longer in this pose (or at least it feels like it)
- On an exhalation round your back and bring your elbow and knee to meet
- Inhale stretch long
- Exhale round your back bringing elbow and knee to meet
- Repeat until you feel done and then do the second side

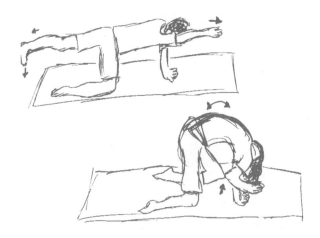

Eagle Armed Sit Ups: Garudasana

- Lay down on yoga mat with feet on the ground
- Cross the right leg over the left
- Place your right elbow under your left
- Hands can rest on shoulders or take the full arm variation where the arms wrap around each other and the palms come to touch
- Take a big inhale, as you exhale bring elbow and knee to touch repeat as many times as you'd like
- Switch sides so the left leg is on top and the left elbow is on bottom. Repeat the same number of times you did on the first side

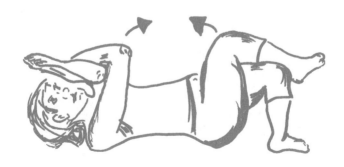

Boat Pose: Navasana

- Begin seated with your sittings bones and feet on the ground and
- Hands hold the back your thighs
- Start to lean back lifting the shins and feet parallel to the ground balancing on your sitting bones
- Stay with your breath here, each exhale connects you to your core strength automatically
- Check in with your shoulders...are they relaxed? Let the shoulders slide down your back away from your ears keeping your collar bone expansive
- If it is easy for you, take the hands away from the legs and extend the legs out making a "v" shape with your body
- You can twisting from one side to the other to strengthen your transverse abdominals

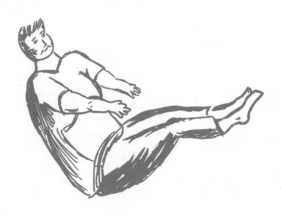

Upside Down Bicycle

- This is a really gentle way to strengthen your core... lay on your back lift your feet off the floor, bend your knees at 90 degrees
- Let your hands rest by your low back, palms facing down
- Start to slowly move your legs as if your were pedaling on a giant bicycle...one that is a few sizes too large
- Stay with your breath
- The slower that you move the more sensation you will notice, imagine you are trudging through thick mud with a heavy old mountain bike
- Flex the feet, spreading toes wide
- Then after awhile, reverse the pedals, going backwards still moving slowly
- After a while, stop and rest
- Stretch your legs long and arms overhead and breathe into your belly

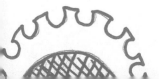
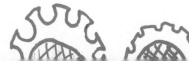

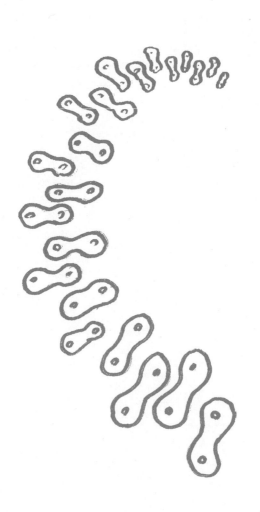

Part 5

Stretch It Out:
Restorative Poses

Restorative poses

Taking time to recover after a long ride is an important part of self care for cyclists. You let your muscles relax after strenuous riding to build strength and replenish your energy for the ride tomorrow. This practice is called an active recovery. You may already know Savasana, which is how you end each yoga session, by laying flat on your back and relaxing into the floor. This is an excellent recovery pose, the most basic of them all.

In this section we explore using props. With this you can use commercial yoga props. If you do not have them or are, say, on bike tour, make do with what is around you. In lieu of a wall, use a tree trunk; instead of a strap use a bike tube or a bungee; and instead of a block or bolster use your rolled up sleeping bag.

Stretches with a strap

Reclining Big Toe Pose: Supta Padangusthasana II

- To begin, lie on your back and use your inhalation to bring your right leg perpendicular to the floor.
- This pose can performed with or without a strap depending on your flexibility. If using a strap place it around the sole of your foot or grab your right big toe and fully extend your leg.
- Pause and breathe into the back of your leg.
- Keep your left heel grounded to the mat and your left arm extended out to the left
- Slowly open your right leg out to the right
- Breathe
- Keep your right leg extended with a very small bend to your knee

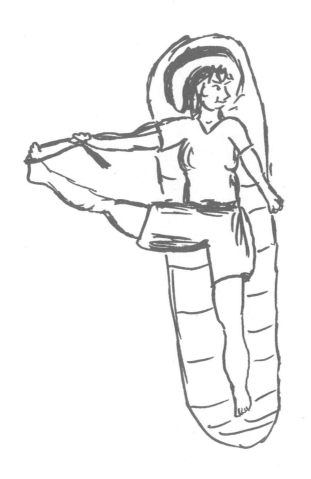

Take it into a Twist...

- Use your core strength to bring your right leg perpendicular to the floor.
- Grab your strap with your left hand (or if you are super bendy your left hand) as you slowly twist your right leg over to the left
- Let your gaze fall to the right
- Each inhale lengthen your spine and each exhale deepen your twist
- Take your time
- Both shoulders root to the ground

This is a very detoxifying twist that feels great in your legs and IT band as well as in your lower back.

Another way to practice this pose is by balancing with your bike. Holding on to your bike brake, stand on one leg and lift the other leg to rest on on your bike rack. This pose requires you to connect with your core and challenges balance. Remember to switch sides.

According to B.K.S. Iyengar in Light on Yoga, this pose offers many benefits to your legs:

"The legs will develop properly by the practice of this asana. Persons suffering from sciatica and paralysis of the legs will derive great benefit from it. The blood is made to circulate in the legs and hips where the nerves are rejuvenated. The pose removes stiffness in the hip joints and prevents hernia."

Stretches with a block

Supported Bridge Pose: Setu Bandu

This supported back bend is great for helping open up the front of your body. I especially appreciate the way this pose feels in my hip flexors.

- To begin, lay on your back with feet on the ground about hip distance apart
- See if your middle finger can barely touch the tip of your heel, this is too see if your feet are close enough to your butt
- Press down through your heels and lift your hips up high
- Gently slide your block under your sacrum, relax your glutes
- Your feet will keep you steady
- Rest into the block
- Breathe
- Stay here as long as you wish

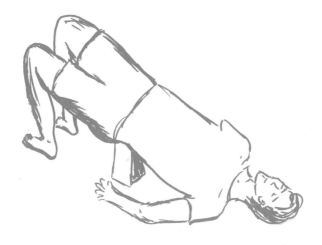

Open Your Heart

One of the most common complaints I hear from bike riders is that their upper back is sore or tight. It is important to counteract the continual rounding of the spine that comes with riding mile after mile. Pause to loosen up your shoulders with gentle shoulder rolls at stop lights. At the end of the day, take time to open up the front of your chest and rest in this pose.

- Position the block so when you lay down your upper back rests on the block
- The top of your shoulders line up with the top of the block, adjust until comfortable
- You may want to put a blanket under your head for support
- Allow your legs to take whatever shape is most natural for you
- Notice how this pose feels
- Stay here as long as feels good
- Focus on your breath and notice where your breath moves in your body
- Keep fingers, toes, and your jaw all very relaxed

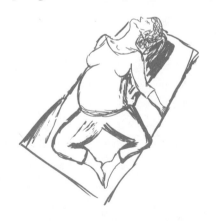

Forward Fold with a Block: Paschimottanasana

This variation of a traditional forward fold allows you to relax the low back and ease into your hamstring stretch.

- Sit on a folded blanket to help maintain the natural curvature of the lumbar spine
- Extend both legs out in front of you
- Feel the sitting bones on the ground
- Sit up nice and tall
- Adjust the block at any height level on your legs
- Hinge at your hips until your forehead reaches the block
- Try flexing and pointing your feet, explore how the feet impact this pose

Another variation of a forward fold is to roll a blanket up and place it under your knees. This will lessen the stretch on your hamstrings and allow you to stretch the low back with a bit of tenderness.

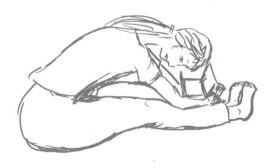

Stretches with the Wall

Reclined Pigeon: Eka Pada Rajakapotasana

- Lay with your back on the ground and your butt a few inches away from the wall
- Place your left foot on the wall, with your knee bent
- Place your right ankle over your left knee and flex your right foot
- If you do not feel a stretch, scoot closer to the wall
- Relax and let the wall do the work
- Breathe deep into your hip
- Switch sides, one hip may be tighter than the other

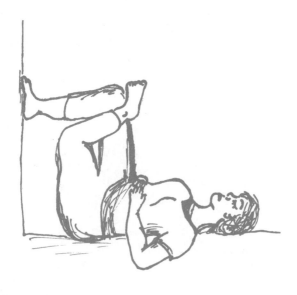

Legs up the Wall: Viparita Karani

- Find a wall to sit beside
- Roll on down onto your back, with your butt is flush to the wall
- Extend your legs up the wall
- If your hamstrings are very tight, you may want to scoot away from the wall a few inches.
- Lie back and relax
- Rest your hands on your belly or by your sides with the palms up
- Relax one muscle at a time with each exhalation, until you melt into the mat.

Legs up the wall pose offers a stretch to the back of the legs without any effort. Let gravity and breath do all of the work. Once fully relaxed, take at least 21 breaths in this pose.

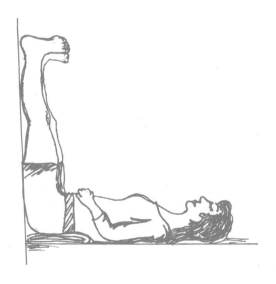

Ninja Death Pose: Eka Pada Rajakapotasana II

Be Warned: this pose was not bestowed the name Ninja Death Pose by yoga teachers for nothing! This variation with the wall is intense, so it is especially important to be gentle and remember to breathe.

It is best to warm-up a little with Chair Pose and Dancer pose first, so the quads are ready to go into a deep stretch. Remember to take your time setting up and getting out of the pose. There should be no pain in your knee or in the front of your leg. If you start to feel even a tiny inkling of pain, gently come out of the pose.

- Place a blanket down to cushion your knee in this pose
- Start on all fours with the feet pressing into the wall
- Step your left foot into a lunge
- Slide the right shin up the wall
- Get your right knee as close to the wall as is comfortable for you, with the knee on the the blanket
- Press your hands into your left thigh and breathe deep down the right side of your body into the quad and hip flexor on the right leg
- Hold several breaths
- Very slowly release the pose and switch sides

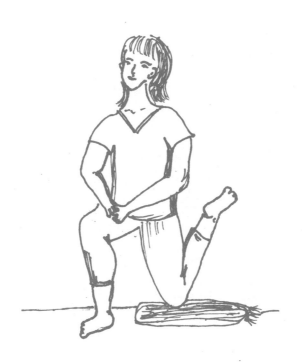

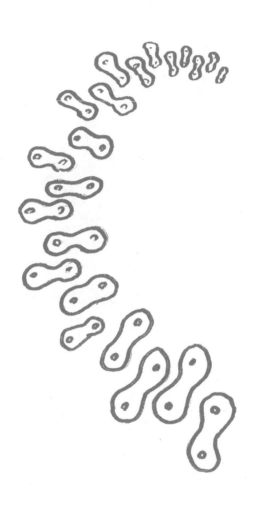

Part 6

Know Your Body:

The Importance of Breath

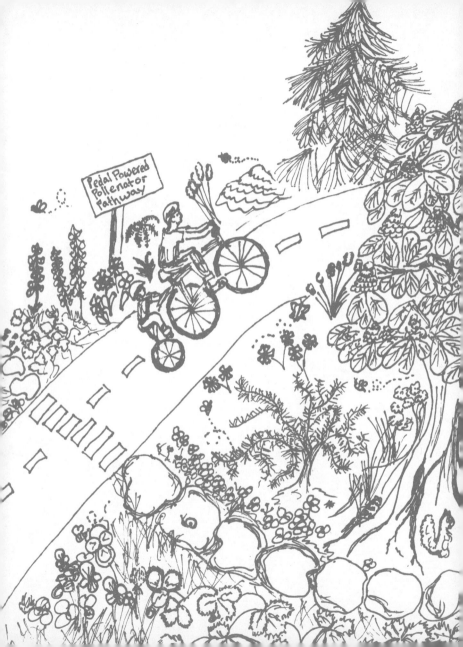

On Breathing

"No individual is independent from the rest of existence. We depend on food for eating, on water for drinking, on space for dwelling, on air for breathing. We depend on Nature every moment. As a matter of fact, the individual is in every way the manifestation of Nature. And there is no distinction between outer and inner nature. The universe is like an organic living tree, and the sun, moon, stars, zodiac signs, humankind, and all creatures are its leaves, flowers, and fruits." - Shri Brahmananda Sarasvati, What is Yoga?

One summer day, I had all of my camping gear on my bike and was riding up a relentless and winding road on Whidbey Island. My breathing— forceful exhalations out of my mouth, followed by full inhalations through my nose—enabled me to channel my power and make it to the top without stopping. It was a variation on a Pranayama technique I learned through yoga.

What sets yoga apart from a variety of other practices is its focus on breath. Yoga literally translates to "yoke" or "union." It is the practice of connecting mind, body and spirit. Our breath is the bridge that connects all parts of ourselves and also connects us to our surroundings. Breath energizes me when I am tired. It is what gave me extra motivation to make it up that last part of that hill before I could coast all the way down to the ferry terminal.

The diaphragm, the key muscle in breath, connects to every vital organ through thick tissues called fascia. When we breathe deep, we access more oxygen. The deeper we exhale, the more stale air we eliminate and the more space we make in our lungs for fresh air.

Our breath is our life force—without it, we die. Each exhale connects you to your core strength and each inhale offers nourishment for every cell in your body. Pause and take a nice deep breath, fully exhale, and see how you feel.

You breathe in the air from pine trees when you ride up a windy, rural road. But what about when you are back in the city? If you ride your bike in traffic with any regularity I am sure you have experienced taking a deep, full-bodied breath just as the truck in front of you expels a dense brown cloud.

This experience is beyond unpleasant, it is toxic. A study on air quality in urban environments from Portland State University notes that "vehicles powered by carbon-based fuels (e.g., gasoline, diesel) have a negative impact on air quality. Vehicular exhaust is the source of a multitude of air contaminants, including particulate matter. The majority of Ultra Fine Particulates (UFP) present in an urban environment are the result of traffic emissions..."

Inhalation of UFPs can lead to a number of health problems related to the cardiovascular system. "The small [size of the UFP] allows for the deepest deposition of particles into the alveolar region of the lungs, pulmonary interstitial spaces, and possible passage into the circulatory system."

I say this not to scare you away from breathing, but to make you more mindful of the bigger picture. There are things we can do to create more breathable air. A study from Beijing shows that when we decrease air pollution we improve our cardiovascular health. Prior to the 2008 Olympic games, the city worked to reduce air pollution by closing down factories and allowing cars to drive on roads every other day. During this time studies showed that the actions taken to clean up the air made an immediate difference in people's health.

A reporter summarized one of these studies this way: "Specifically, they measured blood pressure and looked for blood markers linked to clotting and inflammation—known risk factors for heart disease. They saw big improvements in these measures when the pollution levels went down." After the Olympics, the air pollution and those risk factors both went back up.

I often wonder why more people don't realize how intimately we are connected to our environment. We are permeable beings, and when we inhale we take in what is all around us, no matter where we are. Breath is a cycle that we share with all living things. The oxygen we breathe comes from plants, and when we exhale carbon dioxide the plants breathe it back in. I breathe out, you breathe in, you breathe out, I breathe in. We share the air, just like we share the road.

When I ride my bike in traffic, taking the lane, which happens at some point almost every day, I breathe in these toxic particles. A car emits CO_2 like I do—and it also spews Carbon Monoxide, Hydrocarbons and Particulate Matter to list a few official "hazardous air pollutants" under The Clean Air Act. Because I am riding a bike and using my breath to power my body rather than a V6 engine, I ingest the good air with the bad more directly than my fellow road users.

The PSU researchers warned: "The road user most often traveling through the highest concentrations of UFPs is the urban cyclist. Elevated levels of particles are of concern to bicycle commuters due to the associated health effects and increased respiration and absorption as compared to other road users."

Besides that, I am probably breathing a lot deeper than folks who are barely moving their right ankle to charge up one of Seattle's hills. Maybe they don't even notice the puff of exhaust they leave behind.

In contrast, when I am riding on the Burke-Gilman bike path, I ride past a local brewery and can smell the malted barley. Then a little farther down the path I smell a chocolate factory. (To be fair, there is also a transfer station, a.k.a. a dump, that offers many unpleasant smells to the nostrils.) In mid-spring, residential streets lined with flowering trees emit a magical fragrance, and in late December the smell of pine and cedar fills the air.

Move a little out of the way of car infested lanes and you find a world that is a lot better to breathe in. The PSU study shows that moving cyclist and pedestrian routes away from car traffic contributes to improved air quality on those routes, which contributes to better health.

In Seattle, there is a movement to create routes like this called "neighborhood greenways"—accessible, low-car-traffic pedestrian and bike routes on residential streets. One street in my neighborhood that is being considered for greenway treatment is already part of another project that creates "pollinator pathways." The planting strips along this street have been transformed into pollinator-friendly gardens.

The project website notes that "the Pollinator Pathway is a plan to provide an urban model of support to the foundation of the food web. With a mile-long series of gardens in planting strips...the project establishes a corridor between the two green spaces." It makes sense that these two projects support each other. Pollution caused by high traffic is not only bad for human lungs, but also for pollinators and really for our whole ecosystem. The same things that nurture safe pathways for bees also support safe ways for kids to get to school by the power of their own two feet. Neighborhoods with reduced traffic nurture not only the vitality of our lungs but also the vitality of our communities.

Yoga first drew my attention to the power of breath. Breath is our ultimate tool of transformation: we can shift emotions and thoughts and open even the tightest places in our body. Exhalations detoxify the body. Inhalations bring inspiration. For me yoga and cycling are yoked together by the awareness they cultivate. Yoga brings this inner awareness of breath moving in and out of your body. Cycling is supported by that full breath. Cycling is a way to detoxify our communities and inspire change. Changes manifest in healthier, more active bodies and neighborhoods that are safer and cleaner.

The solution here is to continue supporting cycling, especially by redesigning our urban environments to better accommodate the needs of our lungs. The more people who cycle, the fewer toxins spew out onto our streets. More people biking on neighborhood greenways means more people breathing in cleaner air and more people inviting health into their daily commute.

If we let our breath be our guide, our exhalations are a tool to let go of habits that don't support our vitality. Deep inhalations cultivate the inner strength it takes to pedal through all of our challenges and transform our communities to vital spaces with clean air for all.

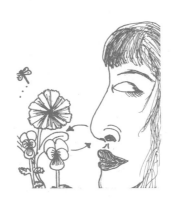

Tips for Working With the Breath

- Begin with observation, notice how you breathe without trying to change it
- Slowly deepen your exhalations, drawing your attention to your diaphragm, remember that the diaphragm contracts on your inhalations pulling in air and relaxes as you exhale, pushing air out of the lungs
- Work gently, take your time and if at any point when working with the breath you are dizzy or light headed, return to a normal, comfortable breath

Observing Your Breath Move

- Place hands on your sides with thumbs facing back and fingers forward between the ribs
- Breathe deep in...and out, feeling your rib cage expand in all directions like an umbrella
- Then try placing your fingers on your mid back with thumbs facing forward to draw your breath in to the back of your lungs

Breathing on Your Bicycle

"Doctor and triathlete John Hellemans recommends that the best breathing for top athletic performance is deep diaphragmatic breathing...Dr. Hellemans also notes the importance of getting into a rhythmic flow with your breathing and synchronizing your breathing with your movement. You can do that by taking a breath when you plant your foot during a stride, when pedaling on a cycle... Find a rhythm and speed of movement that allows you to work within the confines of your breath capacity, so that you are not building up an oxygen deficit." –Donna Farhi, The Breathing Book

Part 7

Seasons of Cycling: Ayurveda

Seasons of Cycling

Cycling connects you very directly to the shifting of seasons. It is huge blessing. You have the chance to notice the first hints of spring, tiny buds forming on trees, flowers popping up through snow. In the fall you are the first to note the shortening daylight. Often bike riding habits take on their own cycles. Each season offers its own highlights and challenges and of course this can be totally different depending on your own bioregion.

We can follow the seasons through ayurveda, an ancient way of looking at health that is also the sister science of yoga. Its foundation is the elements of air, space, fire, water and earth. In the body these elements combine to create three doshas or kinds of energy for different mind/body types: Vata, pitta, kapha. Vata is a blend of air & space. Pitta is fire and water. Kapha is water and earth.

Each person has their own unique constitution, or blend of the doshas. Usually there is one dominant dosha, but there are some folks who are tridoshic. Your doshas may shift over time and may be exaggerated by the changing seasons.

Here is some advice for rolling with the seasons; the lotus indicates yoga strategies and the wrench indicates bicycle actions.

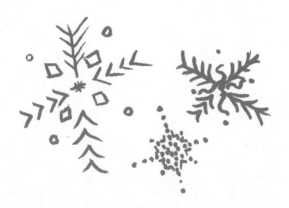

Late Winter - Early Spring (Kapha)

Be thankful for your bike in winter. Even as grey rainy days seem to go on forever, it important to maintain your own inner fire. Everyone has their own personal method for coping with dark days and chilly weather.

In the winter months, year round cyclists can practice the habit of non-judging. Rather than assuming biking in the rain or snow is terrible, start to pay attention to the sensations. Dig deeper, notice the warmth that emanates from your core. Remind yourself of strength, your inner fire, that tapas. If that doesn't work try this mantra: "This is neutral, this is temporary."

Yoga practice is a true delight in winter, it feels good to move, breathe and be active. This is the time of year when kapha energy is abound we want to sink into deep stretches and hang out in restorative poses, while indulging that sometimes is good, it is important in the depths of winter to find your inner fire. Do some core work, or practice hopping into handstand. Try a vigorous vinyasa flow when your energy is feeling low or you are down about the weather. Breaking a sweat will send the winter blues on their way...or at least warm you up.

Late Spring - Summer (Pitta)

There is something about that first evening ride home with no coat, it's like emerging from hibernation. The spring blossoms are in the air and fresh breeze is blowing off of the Puget Sound. Clouds mosey along the evening sky and I can smell spring in the air. It is these moments that folks start to dust off that old bicycle and take to the streets. Pitta is ruled by the element of fire, which inspires people to get moving.

But here is the thing...in summer heat it is easy to overdo it. That is the whole struggle of pitta energy, there is so much drive and ambition, but when left unchecked that leads to burnout and exhaustion. As a remedy for that, on hot days remember to chill out. Find a shady spot under a tree and take Legs up the Tree Trunk. Feel cool grass on your back and let some of that fire go.

There can be a few awkward growing pains if you are starting to ride for the first time or returning after many years. It takes time to acclimate, so remember to be patient and kind to yourself and others. Patience and self-acceptance can be a major challenges for the pitta type who want to be perfect at everything right away.

Late spring and summer are often full of energy. For some people this means they are ready to take their yoga practice into more advanced postures, big backbends like wheel or inversions. This may work well for you, but remember to rest, too.

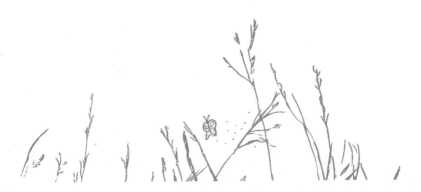

Autumn - Early Winter (Vata)

The blustery winds of fall bring change. As nights grow longer it is important to prepared for the unexpected. Just as squirrels tuck away treats for Winter, cyclists need to start storing more "Just-in-case" gear in your bag.

It is a good time to get a tune-up. Prepare your bike for winter with fenders, bike lights and pack extra layers as the evenings get chilly. I am a huge fan of always having extra socks, gloves and sometimes, a change of clothes. Bike lights become essential—if you can afford it I highly recommend a dynamo hub for the front wheel. The hub converts the energy of your wheel and powers your bike lights. I also like that the lights are bolted on.

It is also important to have enough food to energize you on bike rides. Nothing is worse than realizing your are totally exhausted, starving and five miles away from your destination. Always bring a snack. Even if you end up not eating it, there will be those moments when you are incredibly thankful for them.

Fall is a great time to re-establish a routine. In my weekly classes I start to see the studio fill up with people returning back to the mat. Yoga is an incredibly grounding practice and can help you find a little bit more balance in all elements of your life. In fall, especially around the equinox, I like to focus on balance. Balance is more like a dance with breath. We are always moving, always breathing, balance is not statue still. To have good balance is to dance with pose. Accept the shaking ankle muscles getting stronger as you hold Dancer. To have good balance means sometimes you fall down, but you get up and try again.

What's your dosha?

If you really want to dive into the intricacies of ayurveda, I recommend finding a local practitioner to guide you, but the quiz below will help give you an idea of your bike dosha.

What kind of bike do you ride?
A) Carbon fiber, or something really light and fast
B) Medium build bike with great gear range
C) Solid bike all the way...fat tires and lots of hauling capacity (cargo bikes!)

What is your general riding pace?
A) Fast and in search of new short cuts
B) Move swiftly to the destination
C) Easy going

How do you feel in traffic or surrounded by road rage?
A) Anxious or nervous
B) Irritated and will often yell or react
C) Grounded, calm and courteous

Food is your fuel—what do you like to carry with you?
A) You keep a small snack of trail mix or an energy bar to nibble on just in case
B) You always carry something to eat. If you get hungry you cannot keep riding
C) You'd prefer to pack a full on picnic or stop somewhere to eat

When making a left turn across traffic, you most likely:
A) Just go for it at the first chance
B) Look first and signal, follow all the rules of the road

C) Cautiously wait, maybe using the crosswalk

How much water do you bring with you?
A) Most of the time you've got a water bottle, but sometimes you forget
B) Always have at least one water bottle, if not two or three
C) You carry one, but rarely get super thirsty

What is your stamina on your bike?
A) Short bursts of energy, worn out after long distance
B) Medium stamina
C) Steady, high stamina...you are going the distance

Answer Key
Mostly A = Vata
Mostly B = Pitta
Mostly C = Kapha

See the next page for what that means...

Vata

Think of the element air. Vata is light and cold, like delicate snowflakes in early winter. Vata is quick to move, think and connect. Vata body types are lean, agile and can get cold easily. An air type can be a little flaky, forgetting about that weekly ride they meant to go on or that they need to pump up their tires at least every few weeks. Vata types benefit from warm foods, like soups and stews, that perfect for crisp fall nights. Warming tea, with cinnamon, rosemary and ginger can also help warm and ground airy types.

Vata types may love a light and airy ride, think featherweight wheels and minimalist bikes that integrate cutting edge technology. Vata folks may have some creative short cuts around the city and know some fun people to meet. The only downside is that these riders could be daydreaming as they ride and need a little bit of grounding to keep them focused.

Needless to say that yoga is very helpful in grounding Vata types to the present moment. Meditation and breathing practices may offer a challenge for vata folks, but are a wonderful way to cultivate focus. Paying attention to feet, maybe even taking time for a foot soak with warm water and aromatic herbs after a long day for a delightful dose of self-care.

Pitta

Fire rules pitta, passion, speed and pedal powers these fierce riders. Pitta people have a medium and muscular build, ready to climb hills and take on cyclocross races every weekend. Pitta folks are likely to be fast, strong and competitive. They may be ambitious in many elements of life. Pitta folks may need to avoid spicy food and enjoy fresh salad greens and cooling spices like coriander to tame the fire.

Cycling offers a healthy outlet for fire-filled friends. It is important for Pitta folks to move and be active. Tempers can run high among some pitta people. Remember ahimsa in road rage situations. Patience is definitely a major challenge, like waiting at long stop lights. Pitta folks may be major advocates for cycling.

A yoga practice may invite a little relaxation into the regular routine. While pitta types might be drawn to the most vigorous yoga classes they can find, chances are a Yin or restorative yoga class would serve their stress levels better. Also Pitta folks usually have enough internal heat and can skip heated yoga classes.

Kapha

Think of Earth, in particular mud. Earth met with water, a nourished and strong constitution, kapha folks are solid and caring individuals. They provide stability and grounding to those around them. Kapha types tend to prefer salty and sweet foods. It is important to balance out those tastes by including astringent or bitter flavors into the palate. In early Spring some great bitter greens start emerging from the ground. These fresh plants like spinach, arugula and mustard greens offer important nutrients to energize your ride.

Kapha cyclists would prefer to go the slow, safe and steady route. Kapha types are likely to be well prepared for the weather, with ample lights for visibility and probably a rear-view helmet attachment. Kapha folks might be major proponents of safe routes to schools to make sure everyone they love can bike around the neighborhood safely.

Yoga reminds kapha folks that change is always happening and that a little flexibility helps us all. Kapha folks may change their mind slowly, preferring to stay consistent rather than change, so it is important to find a regular practice to build upon.

Whatever your dosha...

Follow your instincts and do what feels right for you. There are many types of yoga, from the heated and vigorous to the restorative and calming. It may take a few classes at different locations, times or teachers to find the right fit. The same thing goes for bicycles. Sometimes it is all about speed or cargo capacity, but as I am just learning now, it is ok to try and use different bikes. If you don't like your bike, sell it and find one that really fits your life. Celebrating the great diversity of yoga and bikes means that you can experiment and learn what is appealing to you.

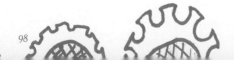
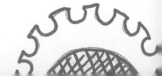

Interlude

Ghost Flats

The other day I was biking home and decided, like I most often do, that I would prefer the slightly longer, windy road that leads up the backside of the hill. I am drawn to the winding curves of the switchback road instead of a beeline straight up. It is also home to one of my favorite spots in Seattle, the Louisa Boren Denny memorial stone on Interlaken Blvd.

In the 1890's City Engineer George F. Cotterill was scouting out good routes for bikes and buggies. Interlaken was established as the primary route between Capitol Hill and Lake Washington. This road was specifically designed with cycling in mind, as well as to capture splendid views. It was these bike routes that laid the foundation for the city's Boulevards. In 1913 the adjacent park was named after Louisa Boren Denny, the last remaining pioneer from the Denny Party, the white folks who "founded" Seattle.

About midway up the hill there is a memorial stone placed to honor Louisa by the Washington Women's Pioneering Organization. I've always been drawn to the that stone and not only because it is a great place to stop for a water break. This admirable pioneer woman was interested in a variety of subjects including philosophy, chemistry and botany.

Legend has it that she brought her beloved sweetbriar rose bush all the way from Illinois to Seattle. The lovely and aromatic rose can be found growing along the shores of the Puget Sound today.

Riding a bicycle on these historic routes connects to me to the history of this place and the Pacific Northwest plants surrounded the streets. And in summer I love to nibble on the blackberries fighting to claim roadspace. They are not the native variety, but I guess me, Louisa, and the blackberry and all have that in common. Part of what makes riding a bike so wonderful is I can take the most beautiful routes around town. Instead of fighting through the traffic downtown and taking the (albeit very nice) buffered bike line across the bridge to run errands, I can cut through the park and take the bike path.

In the dark moonless nights riding on the crumbling road stirs sound of an impending flat tire. You stop to check, but alas your wheels are fully inflated. So you ride on, but the sound of ghost flats will haunt you until you reach the top of the hill. It is like riding in the tracks of all the people who have biked here before you.

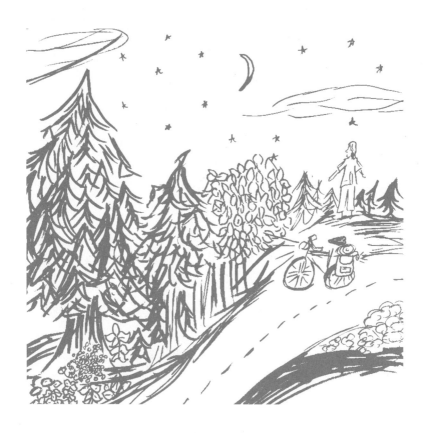

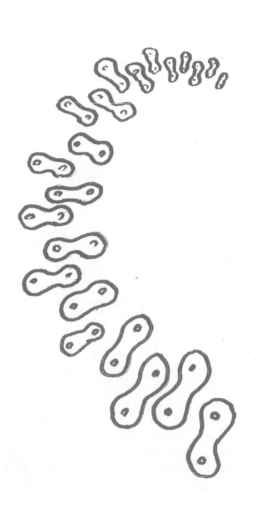

Part 8

Spinning Wheels of Energy: A Chakra Guide

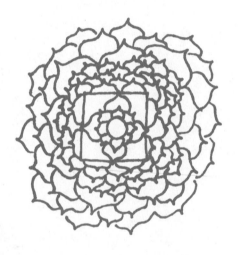

A basic guide to chakras for you and your bike

Tools are integral in unlocking the secrets of your body and your bicycle. Allen wrenches, a third hand (either the tool or a good friend), and a guide (be it intuition, a book, or a mechanic) are all good tools to help you repair and enhance your bicycle. Yoga is a tool to cultivate a strong, flexible body and a calm mind.

Chakras, one aspect of yoga, offer great insight for deepening your understanding of your body. Chakra translates to "disk" or "wheel." Chakras are like spinning wheels of energy inside the body, propelling us forward through time and space. The seven primary chakras are located along the spine. Each chakra also relates to specific developmental processes in our bodies. For example the root chakra addresses the most basic needs of food and shelter, while the third-eye chakra relates to vision.

As I learned to work on my bike I began to see similarities between ways you maintain your bike and your chakras. First, you have to get out the gunk, dirt, stress, tension, anger, apathy or whatever is holding you back. Then you need to invigorate it with new life, energy, grease, air, or lube. It takes time and a little work to get things balanced. And it always seems that once you have one kink worked out, you find something else that needs tuning up.

The lower chakras are more physical and tangible and relate directly to specific bike parts. The upper chakras relate to the intangible aspects of cycling. Start working from the ground up. When learning bike maintenance, you start with the flat tire and then work up to overhauling the headset. When exploring your chakras, begin in a comfortable seat, start from the base of the spine and work up to the crown of your head.

To assist you in your explorations I have included a meditation to try and action items for each chakra. The lotus indicates a yoga-based action and the wrench a bike-based action.

Root Chakra

Muladahara, the root chakra, is located in the perineum and relates to our most basic physical needs, like food and security. Its element is earth and its color is red like blood, birth, or beets.

Each chakra is associated with a particular right. The root is "The Right to Be Here." For cyclists, this chakra is about the right to take up space on the road. A stable connection to the earth helps us feel secure and grounded. The base of the spine connects to the seat, and it is here where we rest into our bicycles. Bicycles root to the ground with their tires—the bike's foundation.

The shadow of this chakra is fear. Fear can inhibit folks from riding a bike in traffic. Learning alternative routes and riding with a friend are good ways to overcome initial anxiety.

Take Action

 We need grounding most often after being shook up or stressed out. Spills, honks and close calls happen—when they do, take a moment to check in with your body. Stop and notice the ground below you. What parts of your body touch the earth? Find a spot to lay down on the ground or a place to sit with your back supported by a bench or tree. This will calm your nervous system and allow your heart rate to stabilize. Notice your breath. Completely exhale and slowly deepen your breath. Check in with how you feel. Take care of immediate needs like hydration or bike repair. Ask for help if you need it.

Ride a bike you feel comfortable on. If you need more support, switch to wider tires or adjust your seat. Learning simple bike maintenance, like fixing a flat tire will help you feel more prepared for the unexpected. Your local community bike project or co-op should have free or affordable maintenance classes. You can also learn from a book or check out the vast number of videos online.

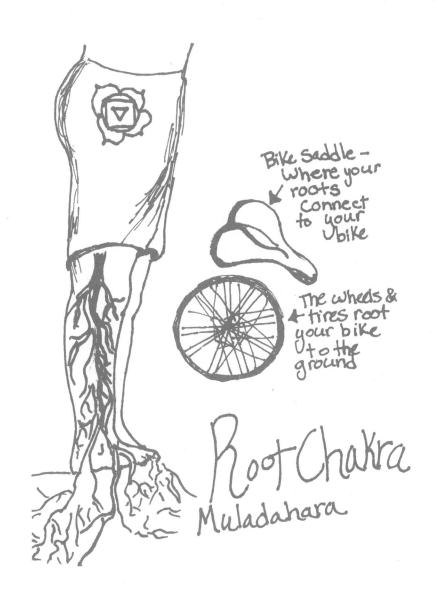

Bike Saddle – Where your roots connect to your bike

The wheels & tires root your bike to the ground

Root Chakra
Muladahara

Sacral Chakra

Savdhistana, the sacral chakra, translates to "sweetness." The second chakra is located by the sacrum, the triangular bone in the lower back near the base of the spine. It is represented by the vibrant color orange and the element water.

The root chakra keeps us rooted and stable; our sacral chakra sets us free. It represents the beginning of our mobility, like the first day you rode a bike all by yourself. Here duality is introduced: We have both stillness and movement, effort and ease.

This chakra embodies the sweeter elements of life. Explore the world with passion and excitement. You have the right to feel your body move, to let go and coast down the hill and feel the sweat on your skin. On a bicycle, this chakra is the hub and the wheels, where movement stems from.

The sacral chakra is about momentum, bike-sexuality, and the joy ride. It's the feeling of the fresh air on your skin and your heart beating as you bike with your sweetie to a serene lookout.

Take Action

Standing with feet parallel and a little wider than your hips, turn your attention to your hips, pelvis and lower back. Make small circles with your hips as if hoola-hooping, then go the other direction. Shake your booty! This will release any built up tension in the hip joints. Do a little dance, laugh, and have a good time.

Enjoy the beauty of the bicycle wheel. It is a mandala, which in sanskrit translates to "wheel" and is an image used for meditation. Lacing the spokes of a bike wheel is a meditation in which you take static parts to make a dynamic whole that is capable of movement. True your wheels and repack your hubs to feel more freewheeling in life.

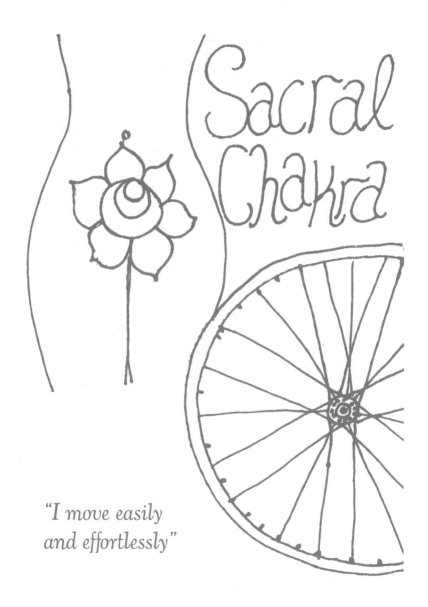

Sacral Chakra

"I move easily
and effortlessly"

Solar Plexus Chakra

Manipurna or "lustrous gem" relates to our ego, will, and drive. Its color is yellow like the sun.

It is no wonder that this chakra relates to the drive train. It is through our pedals and gears that we can go faster and sprint up hill. We are transformed by the awareness or our own power, the knowledge of being strong enough to bike to work or do a handstand.

The solar plexus is our third chakra, where we learn the right to take action and show off our uniqueness to the world. Our lustrous gem shines bright like fire, and like that burn we feel in our legs as we pedal to our limits. Carbohydrates are the food group of this chakra— good fuel for the fire.

Take Action

With the solar plexus it is important to find your edge, the place where you are growing without overextending yourself. If you tend to be a slower cyclist, bike as fast as you can every once and awhile and see how long you can sprint. If you always ride your fastest, try slowing down on a scenic road. How slowly can you pedal without falling over? Core strengthening exercises like sit ups, boat pose, and fierce pose are another way to support the solar plexus chakra.

Lube your chain and get that gunk out of your drivetrain to invite action into your life. For some reason when you lube your chain, all of a sudden it seems you can ride three times faster than before.

Pedal with all your Power

Solar Plexus Chakra

Heart Chakra

Anaharta literally means "unstruck" or "unbroken." The heart chakra, of course, relates to love and compassion.

Your bicycle's heart chakra is in the headset and extends to the handlebars. The headset is hidden in your bike, and keeps you centered. Your heart chakra is protected by your rib cage and is the center of your chakras, connecting the lower chakras with the upper chakras.

Our hands are an expression of the heart—touch is one way we communicate compassion. We use our hands to steer and brake; we can challenge our sense of balance and trust when we ride a bike without hands. My bike fixin' friend noted that the reason you can ride without hands is because you have a headset to keep you balanced.

The heart chakra also captures riding for the love of it, like when someone offers you a ride home home but you would rather bike.

Take Action

Keep your heart open. Slide your shoulders down away from your ears when you ride your bike. This posture facilitates deep, full breathing and keeps your heart forward. Ride with your heart full of compassion and aspire to see other people on the road as humans rather than obstacles in your way.

Are your hands comfortable when you ride? If they are not, try adjusting your handle bars and brake levers and even replacing your grips to find a comfortable spot for all of your fingers.

Heart Chakra

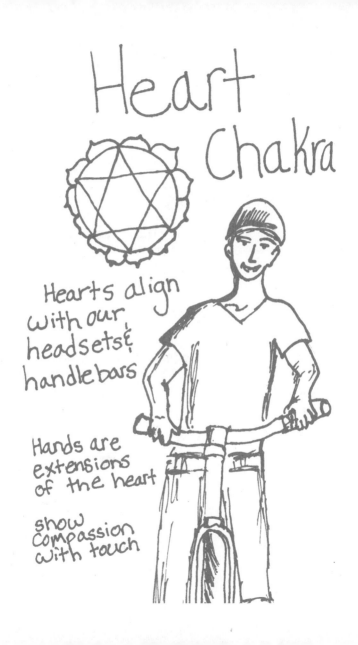

Hearts align
with our
headsets &
handlebars

Hands are
extensions
of the heart

show
Compassion
with touch

Throat Chakra

Vissuddha means "purification" and is related to creativity and expression. The element is sound and relates to our sense of hearing.

On a bicycle, the sounds of the streets inform you of your surroundings. I can hear when a car is coming up behind me or notice the sounds of birds flying overhead. We communicate on our bikes with our voice or our bells, letting others know we are coming up behind them, or just saying hello!

Cycling advocacy and activism are related to this chakra. When we organize a group ride or work to make safer streets, we are using our "Right to be Heard." Our voice is also linked to creative expression and inventing your own interpretation of cycle chic.

Take Action

Practice listening to what is around you in a variety of environments. Stop in a park, notice the sounds near highways and train tracks. Notice the sounds of other bicycles, dogs barking and wind blowing. Practice really listening to other people when they are talking.

There are lots of ways to communicate clearly as your ride your bike. Put a bell on your bike, organize a ride, call a politician to support bicycle initiatives, say "hi" to other people.

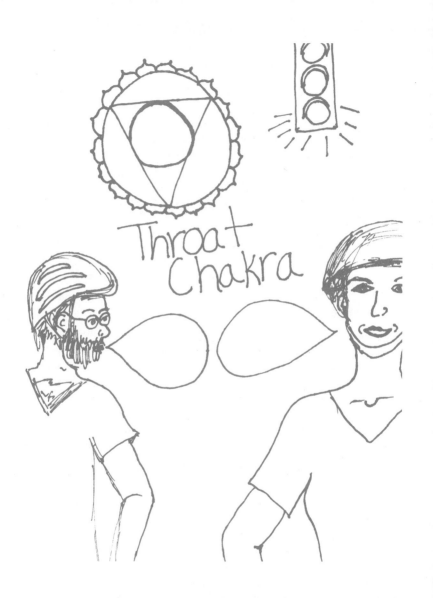

Throat Chakra

Third Eye Chakra

Ajna means "to perceive." It comes as little surprise that the third eye chakra relates to sight and vision. The color for this chakra is violet or indigo, the color of dark nights.

We can see thanks to light. Your bike light illuminates your path at night. In this chakra we find the right to see the outer world and also to cultivate our minds' eye through imagination and intuition. We can transform visions that dwell in imagination into reality.

Strengthen your intuition as you ride your bike by listening to it and heeding your first impressions. Trusting your intuition is imperative as you ride, especially when exploring new places.

Take Action

 Peripheral vision is important for scoping out traffic and noticing cool street graffiti. To increase your field of vision try this exercise: Gently turn your head to the left and right, noticing how far you can see. Then turn your head to the left but look right and then switch. Repeat slowly twice more on each side. Then look to the left, look to the right, and see if your vision has expanded! Please practice this yogic eye exercise while seated on the ground and not while riding.

Take a map and explore a part of town you've never biked to before. Pay attention to colors, plant life, buildings, people's faces, birds, art, and everything else.

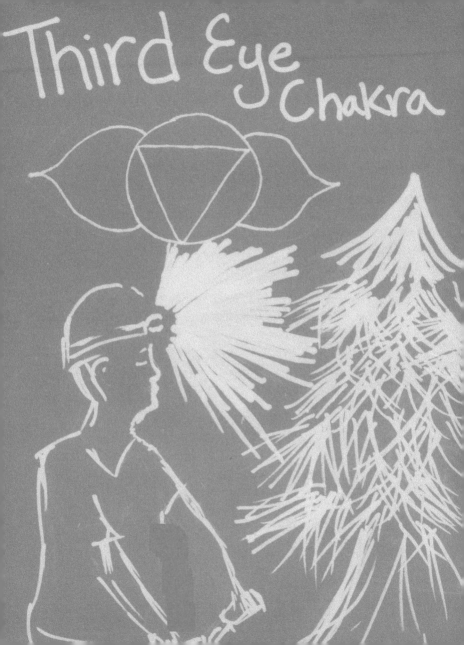

Crown Chakra

Sahasrara means "thousandfold lotus" and relates to thought, understanding and bliss. The aptly named crown chakra exists at top of your skull and extends above your head. While our roots anchor us to the earth, the crown reaches to the sun.

The crown chakra relates to our brain, our internal operating system. How we think and perceive things creates our understanding of the world. Riding a bike alters the way you navigate through neighborhoods and cities.

A mental shift accompanies the transition from driving to biking. Many car oriented folks are baffled by the fact that someone could ride a bike for forty minutes to a party. Instead of viewing it as a chore, I see it as an opportunity for adventure with a group of friends.

On my bicycle, the world is my teacher. We have the right to know we are a part of something much bigger than ourselves. Cycling integrates us with our whole urban environment. On a grand scale, it reminds us that we are fully enmeshed with the seasons and the web of life. Magic exists within the kinetic energy of this simple machine.

Take Action

 Consider your bike ride to be a moving meditation. Notice all the sensations: Air on skin, steady breath, sweat rolling down your brow. Move with keen awareness of your body and surroundings. Obstacles will arise and you will be swept out of that steady, calm mind. When that happens, just return your focus to your breath. Your breath is always present!

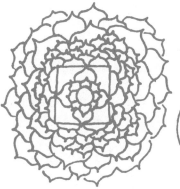

Crown
Chakra

The
world
is my
teacher

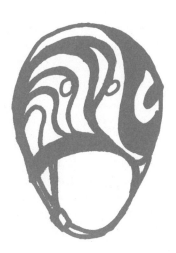

Chakra Meditation

You may notice you have greater reactions to or awareness in some chakras and less in others. Please remember that chakras are a tool for gathering information on how you work and feel. There is no right or wrong way to work with your chakras.

- Find a comfortable seat and take several deep breaths
- Shut your eyes, let your hands rest on your lap and find a tall spine...breathe
- Begin with the root chakra and go up the spine to the crown
- Imagine the color of each chakra and its location in your body
- Chant the sound, whisper and think the sound for that chakra three times each
- Take a moment to notice what is present before continuing up the spine
- After you reach the crown slowly go down the spine back to your root chakra.

These are the chakras' names, locations, colors, and sounds for your meditation:

Root chakra, perineum, red, LAM
Sacral chakra, lower back, orange, VAM
Solar plexus chakra, under the ribs, yellow, RAM
Heart chakra, sternum, green, YAM
Throat chakra, neck, blue, HAM
Third eye chakra, between eyebrows, indigo, OM
Crown chakra, top of head, white, silence

Meditative Bike Maintenance

Can you find the zen of adjusting your fender bolts? It may take focused ujayii breathing, in and out of the nose with gentle constriction in your throat, to find enough focus to get your derailleurs perfectly aligned. I often struggle with keeping my cool while working on my bike, but it helps to check with my breath and pay attention to my body's alignment.

Conclusion

Both riding a bike and doing yoga are activities that we can do alone and together. Practicing alone offers us a personal journey of discovering new places in your body and on the streets. Yoga and cycling infuse me with personal power, connecting me to the strength I contain. When we get together and all attend the same group ride or class, we build more than personal strength—we strengthen our connections with each other. We can use these tools together to develop the grace and flexibility to invite meaningful change into our communities.

Keep on pedaling, stretching and breathing.

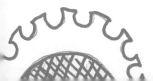
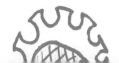

Glossary

Anatomy Stuff

Agonist (AKA Prime Mover): The muscle that is doing the most work, in any movement

Antagonist: The muscle that counteracts the agonist, while the agonist contracts the antagonist will extend

Distal: Closer to the hands and feet; opposite of proximal

Insertion: Where the muscle ends, always distal

Fascia: Thick connective tissue that surrounds all muscles, fascia helps us keep our shape. It is most prominent in the IT band, which can commonly aggravate long term bike riders. Remember it takes holding a posture at least 3 minutes to stretch the fascia, not just the muscle.

Ligaments: Connect bone to bone

Origin: Where the muscle begins, always proximal

Proximal: Closer to the trunk of the body, opposite of distal

Sacrum: Triangular bone at the base of the spine that creates stability in the pelvis

Synergists: Muscle groups that assist the Agonist in a movement

Tendons: Connect muscles to bones

Yoga Stuff

Asana: Sanskrit word that translates to "a comfortable seat;" the term used to describe yoga poses

Ashtanga: The eight limbs of yoga, or the yoga disciplines as B.K.S. Iyengar calls them:

"The yogic disciplines are yama (restraint) and niyama (practice or observance). These disciplines channel the energies of the organs of action and the senses of perception in the right direction. Asana (posture) results in balance, stillness of mind and the power to penetrate the intelligence...Pranayama (control of energy through restraint of breath) and pratyahara (withdrawal of the senses) help [one] explore the hidden facets and enable [one] to penetrate to the core of being. Dharana (concentration), dhyana (meditation) and samadhi (total absorption) are the fulfilment of yogic discipline."

Bandha: Sanskrit word that translates to locks; there are three bandhas in the human body; the pelvic floor, the lower belly and the throat. The pelvic floor or Mula (Root) Bandha draws energy up from the legs into the pelvis. The Uddiyana Bandha is two fingers under the belly button; physiologically this is where you spinal cord connects to all the major nerves that go down to the feet. To engage this bandha think of pulling your belly button closer to the back of your body and up towards your ribs. Engaging this lock while riding will aid in efficiently using your leg strength and protect your lower back. The third, Jalandhara Bandha, is in the throat.

Chakra: Wheel or spinning disk, chakras are energy centers throughout your body. The easiest way to access the feeling of chakras is by closing your eyes and rubbing hands together and then slowly pulling palms apart. The swirling sensation is the energy from the chakras in the hands.

Niyama: These are the best practices guides on how to stay in a good relationship with life. Seek cleanliness, contentment, discipline and get to know yourself and let go of the need to control everything.

Mudras: Gestures, the yoga of the hands. Many mudras come very naturally. Practicing different mudras can also be a great form of meditation. Try sitting with your hands resting palm up on your knees. Bring your thumb to meet your pointer finger in each hand. Then release. Continue by connecting your thumb to each of your fingers. Move slowly and stay in touch with your breath.

Ujjayi: A breathing technique where you breathe in and out of the nose; sometimes called the "Ocean Breath" because it sounds similar to waves of the ocean echoed in seashells. The word translates to "victorious breath," because it cultivates the focus in your body and mind. This is a great breath for a yoga class; however, on a bicycle riding up a large hill or a hauling a heavy load it is too warming. When you are are feeling overheated, exhale out of your mouth.

Vinyasa: My favorite sanskrit translation for vinyasa is "to place in a special way." At many yoga studios a vinyasa is a string of poses that flow from one pose right into the other, usually a plank pose to backbend and back to downward facing dog, with room to embellish or simplify. The key thing to a vinyasa is to move with your breath leading the way.

Yama: The yamas are yoga's "do not" list of behaviors. Don't be mean, don't lie, don't steal or go too crazy with sex, drugs and rock and roll. Finally, don't hoard stuff you don't need.

Bike Stuff

Derailleurs: The parts of the bike that shift the chain from one gear to another, by derailing the chain from its path.

Drivetrain: This is a collection of all the components on the bike that make your bike pedal and change gears. This includes: The bottom bracket, the crankset, the pedals, the chainring, the chain, the derailleurs and the cassette.

Headset: This is the component of the bike that provides the ability to turn, the headset rests in the head tube of the frame and the fork.

Hub: The center of the wheel that holds the axle and with the bearings that magically make the wheel spin.

Fenders: This useful component protects you from the road gunk and rain sprayed up by your wheel. Fenders come in a variety of styles, sizes and made of many materials like metal, plastic or wood.

Frame: This is the main body of the bicycle and it is important that your frame fits you. Be sure you can comfortably stand over the top tube of your frame. There is some variation of materials for frames but the most common ones are metal, but bamboo is starting to emerge as a viable source of locally grown bike frames...

Overhauling: The process of taking apart a hub and adding new grease and sometimes new bearings.

Panniers: Originally panniers were French undergarments, those 18th century side hoops that go under skirts. I imagine that they were not very comfortable for women to wear. In the bike world though, panniers are bags or baskets that frame either side of the rear rack. They are incredibly useful for carrying all kinds of stuff and are much better for your spine than a backpack.

References & Further Reading

Clark, Ethan, and Shelley Lynn Jackson. The Chainbreaker Bike Book: A Rough Guide to Bicycle Maintenance. Microcosm, 2010. Print.

Farhi, Donna. The Breathing Book: Good Health and Vitality through Essential Breath Work. Henry Holt, 1996. Print.

Horton, Carol A., and Roseanne Harvey. 21st Century Yoga: Culture, Politics, and Practice. Kleio, 2012. Print.

Iyengar, B.K.S. (1975) Light On Yoga. Schoken Books.

Iyengar, B.K.S. (1993) Yoga Sutras of Patanjali. Omnia Books

Judith, Anodea. Eastern Body, Western Mind: Psychology and the Chakra System as a Path to the Self. Berkeley, CA: Celestial Arts, 2004. Print.

Koch, Liz. The Psoas Book. Guinea Pig Publications, 1997. Print.

Long, Ray, and Chris Macivor. The Key Muscles of Yoga: Your Guide to Functional Anatomy in Yoga. Bandha Yoga Publications, 2006. Print.

Gratitudes

Thank you to everyone who helped make this book possible. Especially my family for teaching me how to ride a bike and supporting me as I pedal down my own path. Thank you to my partner Tom Fucoloro for love and inspiration. Thank you to my wonderful publisher and mentor Elly Blue for nurturing my ideas. Thank you to my mentors in yoga and all of my teachers.

I would like to thank everyone who donated to the Kickstarter campaigns or purchased the first edition. Without you this book would be a series of thoughts and doodles rather than something tangible.

About the Author

Kelli Refer lives in the hilly city of Seattle. Her childhood love of bike riding was rekindled as an adult in 2008, when she turned in to a full time bike commuter. She has been an avid practitioner of yoga since 2005 and has been teaching since 2009 after earning her 200 hour Registered Yoga Teacher certificate.

Her other passion is botany and learning about the plants of the Pacific Northwest that she discovers on bicycle tours. And she can't get enough of practicing yoga on beaches, in forests, and in bike lanes.

You can find more of her writing about the joy of bicycles and yoga on her blog at pedalstretchbreathe.com and follow her on Twitter at @yogaforbikers.

Pose Index